It's All in Your HEAD

And Also Your Neck, Back, and Gut

It's All in Your HEAD

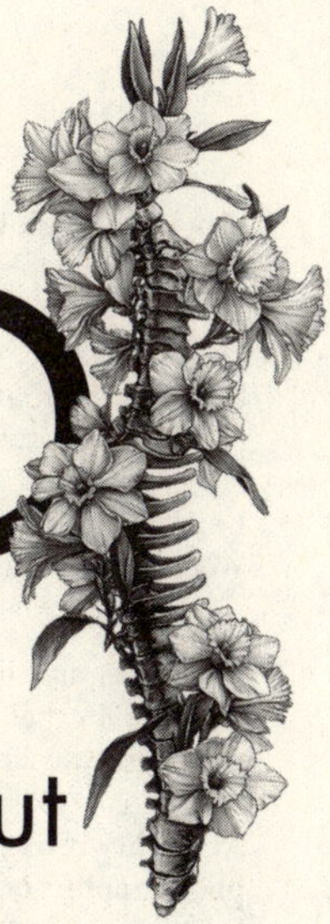

And Also Your Neck, Back, and Gut

how beliefs and emotions sneak into the body, why it matters, and how we can ***heal***

Dr Shalini Poddar

HAY HOUSE

HAY HOUSE INDIA
New Delhi • London • Sydney
Carlsbad, California • New York City

Hay House Publishers (India) Pvt Ltd
Muskaan Complex, Plot No. 3, B-2, Vasant Kunj, New Delhi – 110070, India

Hay House LLC, P.O. Box 5100, Carlsbad, CA 92018-5100, USA
Hay House UK Ltd, 1st Floor, Crawford Corner, 91-93 Baker Street, London W1U 6QQ, UK
Hay House Australia Publishing Pty Ltd, 18/36 Ralph St., Alexandria NSW 2015, Australia

Email: contact@hayhouse.co.in
Website: www.hayhouse.co.in

First published by Hay House India, 2025
10 9 8 7 6 5 4 3 2 1

ISBN 978-93-6611-342-5
ISBN 978-93-6611-718-8 (Ebook)

Printed at Replika Press Pvt. Ltd.

FSC
www.fsc.org
MIX
Paper | Supporting responsible forestry
FSC™ C016779

Hay House is committed to a sustainable future for our business, our readers and our planet. This book is made from Forest Stewardship Council® certified paper.

I dedicate this writing to all my teachers, clients, and loved ones whose journeys and wisdom have deepened my understanding of the beautiful connection between body and emotions.

CONTENTS

Preface

When working in therapy, there are many aspects to consider, ranging from ethical factors such as confidentiality to theoretical ones, like choosing the appropriate approach or technique for each case. Yet, one foundational pillar of therapy that is rarely emphasised in these discussions is the art of case conceptualisation.

Case conceptualisation is essentially the initial assessment of a new client, accompanied by a preliminary plan for future sessions. It involves recording all relevant information about the client, starting with the issue they have come to therapy for, any other difficulties they are currently facing, and the various factors that may have contributed to or are maintaining the presenting issue. The therapist gathers this information through interviews, observations, and assessments, noting the interventions used or planned, and keeping track of outcomes and follow-up sessions. This method of documenting relevant information enables both the therapist and client to gain clarity about the issue at hand, identify potential triggers that might impact recovery, and monitor the course and effectiveness of therapy. It serves as a dynamic record of what occurs during sessions and how the client progresses over time.

One of the simplest and most widely used conceptualisation frameworks is the Four Ps Model, which organises the case information into four categories: predisposing, precipitating, perpetuating, and protective factors. This model is often paired with a concept map, which provides a visual representation of how these elements are interconnected and how they affect the client in different ways. This framework functions as a road map for the therapeutic journey, one that is regularly updated and refined in collaboration with the client.

Below is a sample of how the Four Ps are typically mapped.

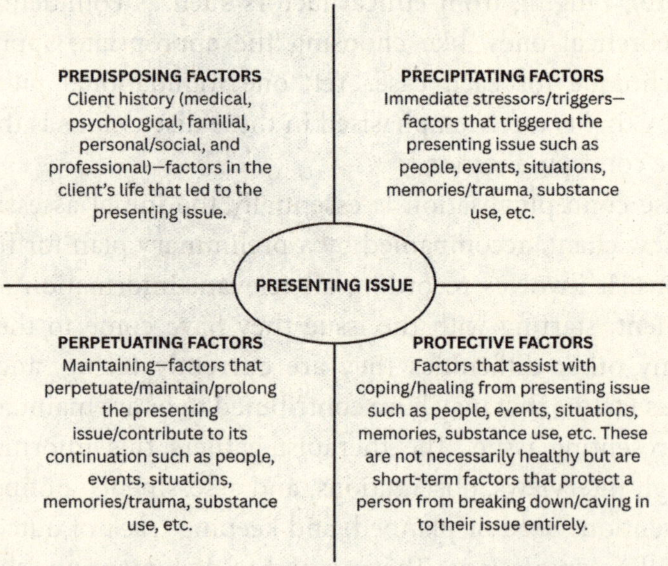

Over time, several other models for case formulation have been developed. Two commonly used methods are the PAIP and SOAP formats. Let's take a closer look at each of them.

1. PAIP Method

The PAIP method stands for Problem, Assessment, Intervention, and Plan. The therapist begins by recording the presenting problem, i.e., the primary concern that brought the client to therapy and is typically the focus of the session. They then make an assessment of the client, which may include general observations about the client's mental, emotional, and physical state, behaviour patterns, and notable habits. Following this, the therapist records the interventions used during the session, along with those planned for future work. These can range from the broader therapeutic approach (e.g., psychodynamic or gestalt) to specific techniques like the empty chair or guided imagery. Finally, a treatment plan is developed in collaboration with the client, outlining goals, planned interventions, observed results, homework, and follow-up steps.

2. SOAP Method

The SOAP method stands for Subjective, Objective, Assessment, and Plan. Like PAIP, this approach involves documenting the client's presenting concerns, therapist observations, and a future plan. However, SOAP introduces two distinct observation categories: subjective and objective. Subjective observations include the client's own words and perceptions, often recorded through direct quotes during sessions. Objective observations, by contrast, refer to what the therapist notices, such as the client's body language, tone, or affect. The assessment here is the therapist's clinical impression of the client, combining subjective and objective elements.

The choice of method depends on the therapist's personal style—how they prefer to organise case notes—as well as the purpose the case files serve. For instance, files might be used purely for internal tracking, or they may be documented as formal case studies for teaching or research.

This book explores the use of these various approaches to case formulation, showing how even abstract client concerns can often be linked to common therapeutic themes. It also demonstrates the value of mapping out a case in a structured way. Each chapter focuses on a specific aspect of the healing process, illustrated through real cases where clients grappled not only with their presenting concerns but also with deeper philosophical questions that arose during therapy. While these issues may appear abstract at first, the case studies highlight how they often reflect broader understandings of human behaviour and how healing can be rooted in sound psychological theory.

Introduction

Body As a Messenger

The body speaks in the poetry of symptoms. A clenched jaw, a gut twisted in knots, an inexplicable heaviness in the chest are not malfunctions or random occurrences. They are messages, like unread letters from your past, written not in words, but in muscle, breath, and pulse. The body remembers what the mind tries to forget, and when words fall short, it speaks on our behalf.

As a hypnotherapist, I have seen how trauma hides in plain sight. One client's sensation of being possessed vanished after she confronted repressed memories of childhood abuse. Another, who had battled chronic fatigue for years, found his energy return within weeks of quitting a job that unconsciously mirrored the emotional neglect he experienced from his father. These aren't supernatural mysteries. They are the biology of belief in action, serving as evidence that emotions buried alive never truly die, but instead live on in the body, waiting to be acknowledged, understood, and released. And when we start to listen—really listen—to the signals of our body, we begin to uncover truths that talk therapy alone might miss. Healing, then, becomes not just a mental exercise but a full-body experience, which involves a remembering, a reclaiming, and an invitation to finally complete a story that has long remained unfinished.

The Aim of the Book

Our journey begins not in the mind but in the body, where stories are not told but stored. Beneath every ache, tight muscle, or restless night often lies an emotional experience or unresolved trauma that the body is trying to express in its own language. While the mind may suppress or rationalise, the body quietly holds the truth.

This understanding invites us to question some of the assumptions of the broader health industry—especially the mental health industry—which still often operates within narrow diagnostic frames. Labels can help, yes, but they can also miss the forest for the trees. What if anxiety isn't a disorder at all, but the body's protest—a fierce, loyal resistance against needs that went unmet for too long? What if your panic attacks are not irrational outbursts, but your body's last attempt to protect an old vow you made when you were too young to put it into words? Vows like 'I must always be perfect,' 'I can't ask for help,' or 'Love must be earned.'

This book explores how such internalised beliefs, silent promises and traumatic experiences can become invisible blueprints etched not just into our beliefs, but into our muscles, our posture, our breathing patterns, even our chronic pain. These embodied imprints govern so much of our adult lives. They influence who we trust, what we tolerate, how we cope, and how we suffer. Remember that your body is not static. It reshapes itself in response to love, rupture, and repair, and each time you pause to notice or give words to what once remained unspoken, you reclaim a part of yourself that has long been waiting to be seen.

What you will find in these pages is not just insight, but a path. This book will act as your translator, offering a new way to understand what your body is trying to say. It will guide you to see your physical sensations, recurring symptoms, and emotional patterns as part of a symbolic language your body has been speaking all along. Each chapter will walk you through the intricate connections between early emotional experiences and adult symptoms, weaving together real stories, therapeutic insights, and practical tools for healing.

You will dive deep into the biology of belief and the psychology of healing. You will learn how the stress you carry today often traces back to formative beliefs, experiences, and promises made in moments of fear or confusion. You will explore how your body holds on to these emotional imprints and, more importantly, how you can begin to safely release them. You will also be introduced to various healing modalities that work with the body and not against it, ranging from somatic therapy and breathwork to body-based mindfulness and energy work. These tools are not meant to 'fix' you, but to reconnect you with the pivotal experiences and parts of yourself that were never broken to begin with—only silenced, suppressed, or misunderstood. Along the way, you will discover that healing is not a formula to follow, but a relationship to build. A relationship with your story, your body, and the version of you that is still emerging.

By the end of this journey, you will begin to read your body's language fluently. You will no longer feel like a stranger to your own nervous system. Instead, you will see each symptom as a sentence in a longer story, one that you now have the power to rewrite. You will understand where your pain comes from, how it speaks, and what it needs to be released.

For those who are new to therapeutic or somatic language, I have presented all topics and concepts in an easy-to-understand, accessible manner. A glossary of key terms is also included at the end of the book for quick reference and clear definitions. You don't need to be an expert to begin. What you do need is curiosity, compassion, and a willingness to listen to what your body has been trying to tell you all along. All in all, this book is not a manual; it is a mirror. Each story, each framework, each exercise offers a doorway, but the journey through it is uniquely yours.

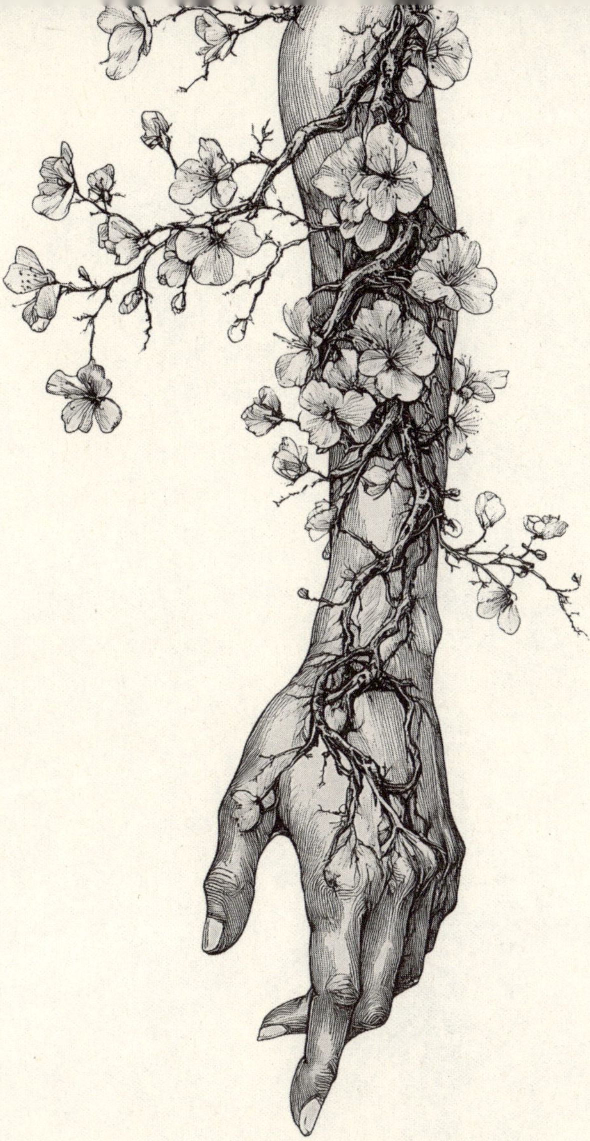

Part I
Awareness and Insight

Chapter 1

WHEN THE BODY SPEAKS

'A body never forgets. It folds grief into shoulders, fear into stomachs, and when the heart has no words, it writes them in pain.'

MOST PEOPLE BEGIN THERAPY BECAUSE OF HOW THEY feel: anxious, low, stuck, overwhelmed. But just as often, they come because of what they are experiencing physically. This might include digestive issues, chronic pain, tension, or recurring headaches that no medical test can explain. In such cases, it is important to notice how the patient's language often reveals the hidden connection between emotion and the body.

- 'My back gives out every time I am under pressure.'
- 'I get this choking feeling whenever I talk about my past.'
- 'I know there's nothing medically wrong, but the symptoms won't go away.'

This highlights the fact that the body has a mind of its own, and in many ways, it does. It responds not only to what is happening now but to the accumulated emotional weight we carry, most of which stems from earlier in life and remains unresolved. These responses may not always appear logical, but they are always meaningful. In other words, the body is not merely the canvas for our symptoms; it is the container for our stories. It stores patterns, sensations, and responses long after a situation has passed, especially if the emotions involved were overwhelming, forbidden, or never fully processed. Over time, when these inner signals are ignored or misread, the body speaks louder. Subtle sensations give way to chronic symptoms. What we call disorders or conditions often begin as the body's attempt to express what the mind cannot yet understand or articulate.

This chapter invites you to begin looking at your symptoms not as enemies, but as messengers. For instance, what if your chronic exhaustion isn't laziness but your body remembering a time when resting wasn't safe? What if your digestive issues are less about food and more about long-swallowed emotions? And in order to begin healing, we must start listening—not just to our thoughts, but to the quiet intelligence of our bodies. Because before a wound is ever spoken, it is first felt.

The Body Keeps Score

When we talk about stress or trauma, we are often referring to experiences that had no room for resolution and the emotional energy that had nowhere to go. It was the fear that had to be swallowed, the grief that was never comforted, and the anger that had to be hidden to stay safe or accepted. These emotions, denied full expression, don't simply vanish. They get lodged somewhere—first in the psyche, and then, inevitably, in the body.

Moreover, we like to believe that if something happened years ago, it stays in the past. But the body doesn't work on the same timeline as the mind. It remembers through sensation, posture, breath, and response. Even when the conscious mind forgets or numbs out an experience, the nervous system can remain stuck in a holding pattern, still waiting for the safety that never came or the release that never happened.

It is important to note that this isn't just poetic language; it is a physiological reality. Research has repeatedly shown how chronic stress and unresolved trauma impact the autonomic nervous system, contributing to dysregulation in breathing, heart rate variability, digestion, sleep, and even immunity. Long-term exposure to emotional strain alters cortisol levels, affects how inflammation is regulated, and rewires brain pathways linked to perception and threat response. Trauma and stress, therefore, are not merely emotional concerns but embodied states. What begins as a psychological wound becomes somatic architecture. Our shoulders hold tension long after the threat is gone. Our gut tightens even when there is no danger. Our breath shortens as if bracing for a blow that never arrives.

So when someone says, 'I carry this in my body,' it is not just a metaphor; it is a neurobiological fact. The body stores what the mind cannot process, and it speaks when words fall short. Over time, if these stored patterns are not understood or released, they solidify into what we call chronic pain, autoimmune conditions, anxiety loops, or even a general feeling of disconnection from the self.

Understanding this helps us move away from blaming ourselves or our bodies and towards curiosity and compassion. Remember, our symptoms are not failures. They are signals from a part of us still waiting to be seen, heard, and healed.

The good news? What has been encoded can be decoded. What has been stored can be safely released. But first, we have to learn to listen.

Learning to Listen

One of the most powerful shifts in healing comes when we move from reacting to our symptoms to truly listening to them. Most of us are conditioned to see symptoms as problems to get rid of. For example, a headache must mean we need a pill, and fatigue must mean we need more coffee. But healing often begins not with suppression, but with attention. It requires a pause, a soft curiosity, and a willingness to ask: What is my body trying to tell me?

This doesn't mean we turn every ache into a complex psychological analysis or overthink every sensation. It simply means recognising that the body is not separate from our emotions, our experiences, or our beliefs. The body is not just a vessel that carries us. Instead, it is a participant in our emotional life. It remembers what the mind forgets and expresses what the voice may never have spoken aloud.

The main takeaway here is simple: When a symptom appears, gently ask yourself, 'When did this begin?' and 'What was happening in my life at that time?' Maybe you won't get a clear answer right away, and that is okay. But the act of asking—of making space for connection—begins the process of awareness.

Over time, patterns may emerge. You might notice how your back tightens every time you feel unsupported. How your jaw clenches when you feel unheard. How your chest gets heavy when you are holding grief. Learn to see your body's responses not as coincidences, but as gentle invitations to explore what lies beneath. Even if no clear cause arises, continue to pay attention. The body communicates in many languages—through pressure, tension, discomfort, heat, tingling, numbness, and even stillness. Each sensation is a doorway, not an obstacle. And as you notice what your body is saying, you can begin to ask: 'What emotion might be connected to this?' Know that you don't need to get it right. This isn't about finding a diagnosis. Instead, it is about developing a relationship with yourself. Curiosity is the goal, not certainty. You are not solving a puzzle; you are listening to a story.

As you practice this over time, something subtle but powerful happens. You begin to notice not just when you are in distress, but when you feel peace. You will begin to identify the people, spaces, and activities that bring you calm, that help you breathe more deeply, that feel like safety. These moments are just as important to your healing as the symptoms are. In fact, they may be even more important.

Always remember that your body isn't trying to sabotage you. It is trying to support you. To protect you. To speak to you in the only language it knows. And when you begin to listen with patience and care, the body often responds—not with silence, but with relief. We will explore this aspect in greater detail in the next section.

Your Body Is Not the Enemy

It is easy to see symptoms as the enemy—something to fix, suppress, or silence as quickly as possible. We are taught to treat discomfort as a disruption, a malfunction, an interruption to our 'normal' lives. But often, symptoms are not the problem. As mentioned earlier, they are the body's language. A subtle—or sometimes loud—attempt to draw our attention to something deeper. To an unmet need. An unresolved memory. A limit that has been quietly crossed too many times.

When we shift from fighting our body to listening to it, something changes. We begin to create the conditions for healing. Not through a magical cure or quick fix, but through presence. Through compassion. Through the recognition that our body is not separate from our story. Rather, our body is the story as it carries the weight of our experiences, our coping patterns, our silences, and our resilience. Every ache, tightness, or chronic condition may be linked to something we have lived through, even if we haven't yet made the connection.

After all, your body has witnessed everything—what you have been through, what you have lost, what you have endured, and how you have adapted. And sometimes, what we experience emotionally but can't express verbally gets stored physically.

This doesn't mean we abandon medical care or stop treating physical illness. It means we stop treating the body like a malfunctioning machine and start relating to it as a wise, sensitive, and expressive part of ourselves. A part that wants to heal, not just function.

As we move through the coming chapters, we will explore how beliefs shape biology, how early childhood experiences shape the way we relate to stress and safety, and how healing isn't always about fixing what is broken, but about understanding what was never allowed to be seen. The body doesn't need to be battled; it needs to be heard.

So for now, consider this simple but powerful question: 'What is your body trying to tell you that your mind hasn't yet allowed you to hear?'

Why Case Studies Matter

Case studies are, perhaps, one of the most insightful tools we have when it comes to understanding the human psyche, not just in terms of behaviour, but in terms of belief, emotion, and meaning-making. While they may not offer the statistical certainty of large-scale research, what they provide instead is depth. They allow us to witness individual stories in all their complexity and nuance.

Through these narratives, we begin to see how personal psychology is never formed in isolation. Each person's engagement with fantasy, belief systems, or emotional coping isn't random; it is shaped by a deeply interwoven web of early experiences, trauma, cultural messaging, and internalised expectations. Additionally, these aren't always loud or dramatic forces. Sometimes, it is the quieter currents—an overlooked childhood need, a repeated family script, or a subtle cultural bias—that shape a person's inner landscape.

For instance, one case may show how a person turns to magical thinking as a way of making sense of chaos in their early environment. Another may reveal how someone internalises guilt and blame because they were repeatedly told to be strong and grateful, even when their emotional world was collapsing. These aren't just stories of dysfunction; they are also stories of human survival. Each adaptation, no matter how puzzling it may seem from the outside, once served a purpose.

What makes case studies even more powerful is their ability to reflect back parts of ourselves. We may not share the same life experiences as the person in the study, but we can relate to the themes: the longing to be understood, the fear of abandonment, the coping strategies developed to feel safe in a world that didn't always feel safe. More importantly, case studies help us understand that emotions and beliefs are not abstract or purely mental; they live in the body. They show us how shame may settle into the chest, how anxiety becomes a constant clenching of the stomach, how the fear of not being enough echoes through one's posture, voice, and choices. These patterns are not imagined; they are embodied. And once we learn to tune into those signs—through awareness, reflection, or therapeutic practices—we can begin to unravel what no longer serves us.

In this way, case studies don't just offer insight. They offer hope. They remind us that these internal narratives are not set in stone. What has been learnt can also be unlearnt. What was once a survival mechanism can, with time and compassion, become a pathway to healing.

By examining these individual journeys with curiosity rather than judgement, we can look inward with the same tenderness and ask: 'What beliefs have I inherited?', 'What emotions have I stored without realising?' and 'What version of the story am I still living, and is it still true?'

Ultimately, the value of case studies lies in their ability to humanise the process of self-understanding. They remind us that we are not alone in our confusion, our coping, or our becoming. And in doing so, they open the door to healing that feels both personal and universal.

In the following section, you will find a case study accompanied by a detailed breakdown. This is intended to help you understand the key themes, perspectives, and patterns to look out for in other case studies presented throughout the book. And don't worry if you come across terms or ideas that feel unfamiliar. Simply note them for now, as we will be covering all key topics and terminology as you progress through the book.

Case Study: Childhood Wounds as Safety Nets

Priya (name changed to protect the privacy of individuals) was thirty-nine when she came to therapy. She was successful, articulate, and deeply tired. She described herself as someone others turned to: 'the calm one,' 'the solid one,' 'the one who holds it together.' But her body told a different story: chronic throat tension, a feeling of choking, a lump in her throat that no scan could explain, and a jaw that locked every night in her sleep. When we traced the origin, we found the moment her voice had been stolen. At twelve years old, she had whispered to her father about the uncle who touched her in ways that made her skin crawl. Instead of shelter, she received a warning. 'Don't ruin our family with lies,' he told her. That was the day her throat first closed. What follows is a layered breakdown of Priya's case, not just as an isolated incident, but as a window into the psychological and physiological imprints of trauma. The sections ahead explore how the body carries unresolved emotions, how symptoms can be understood as survival mechanisms, and how healing involves rewriting these internal scripts.

1. **The Body Maps the Soul**

   Priya's case isn't unique, yet it is remarkable in its physiological precision. Her body had archived the trauma with near-surgical accuracy. The constriction in her swallowing muscles mirrored the way she had learnt to force down her words. The shallow breathing pattern she developed matched the careful control of someone afraid to make a sound. Even her posture told the story: shoulders curled forward, as if still bracing for blame. This was no malfunction. Her nervous system had done exactly what evolution designed it to do. When a child faces unbearable pain, the body steps in to manage what the psyche cannot. The vagus nerve—that intricate web of connection between throat, heart, and gut—became the scribe of her suffering. Where words failed, her flesh spoke. Another important thing to note: the human body remembers what the mind cannot bear to hold. It keeps its own ledger of hurts, etching each unspoken wound into muscle and breath.

2. **The Inner Script and the Body**

   When children consistently encounter certain patterns—being punished for anger, ignored in sadness, or rewarded for suppressing needs—they learn what is allowed and what is dangerous. They begin to script their emotional lives accordingly. 'Always be pleasant.' 'Don't rely on anyone.' 'Keep control or you will get hurt.' This script isn't just mental; it is also physical. A child who had to shrink might now live with hunched shoulders. A child who had to be the fixer might carry jaw tension or digestive issues. In other words, the emotional blueprint lives not just in what we believe, but in how we breathe, move, and react.

3. From Symptom to Survival Strategy

It can be tempting to view emotional patterns as problems to fix. But anxiety, perfectionism, and people-pleasing are not character flaws. They are survival strategies, i.e., responses that once worked, and simply haven't been updated. For Priya, the work of healing began when we stopped treating her throat as a broken part and started listening to it as a witness. Through somatic therapy, we gave voice to what had been silenced. She learnt that the lump was not an enemy to eradicate, but a protest to honour.

As she began to speak her truths in our sessions, something remarkable happened: the constriction eased—not through force, but through being heard. What medicine often dismisses as psychosomatic, I have come to see as the body's deepest wisdom. Put simply, a symptom is never just a symptom. It is a map to places we have forgotten, written in a language older than words. Priya's throat was not failing her. It was reminding her of the girl who still waited to be believed.

4. **The Biology of Survival**

Subconscious vows made in trauma—'I will never trust again,' 'I must be perfect,' etc.—act as invisible fences around joy. These oaths often originate in moments of deep wounding, when survival demands certainty. Left to fester, they can manifest as chronic pain, autoimmune conditions, or self-sabotage. Priya's body also held similar subconscious trauma. Long after the events of her childhood faded from conscious memory, her cells still reacted as if the danger lingered. This was not a metaphor. When we measured her cortisol levels, they told the same story as her clenched throat. It revealed a stress response stuck in perpetual alarm. Science now confirms what therapists have long witnessed. Childhood stress does not simply pass through the body like weather; it embeds itself in biology, elevating lifelong risks for chronic illness and even cellular ageing. It rewrites the very instructions for how to survive, turning our primal defences into our default settings. Priya's choked silence wasn't metaphorical. The moment her father dismissed her truth, her developing brain made two simultaneous recordings. The first was conscious: the shame of not being believed. The second was biological: a flood of stress hormones that etched the lesson into her nervous system. Her amygdala—the brain's sentinel for threat—grew hypersensitive, internalising the belief that speaking up was dangerous. Where others might hear a raised voice and feel momentarily startled, Priya's body reacted as if facing mortal danger. Her muscles tightened, her breath shallowed, and her throat closed. These were not overreactions. They were precise reenactments of a survival strategy that had once kept her safe.

5. **Reconditioning the Script**

The tragedy of developmental trauma is its efficiency. The same plasticity that allows children to adapt to their environments enables suffering to become structural. Neural pathways meant for learning languages get instead trained in vigilance. Stress hormones meant for brief emergencies become a constant background hum. What begins as protection—the freezing, the silence, the perfect obedience—eventually becomes its own kind of prison.

For Priya, the path to healing required more than insight. She needed her biology to learn a new truth. Through somatic work, we helped her nervous system discover that not all authority figures would betray her. That some spaces could hold her anger without collapsing. That a deep breath would not, in fact, summon disaster.

This is the paradox we navigate in trauma therapy. The very systems that once preserved life can later restrict it. Yet the same plasticity that encodes suffering also holds the possibility of its undoing. Each time Priya spoke her truth in our sessions without punishment, each time she noticed her throat relaxing around difficult words, she wasn't just healing psychologically; she was teaching her cells a new alphabet of safety. The body remembers, yes. But it can learn to remember differently.

6. **Rebuilding the Emotional Blueprint**

When early experiences of safety, love, or attunement are missing, the body encodes this as a threat to survival. The child doesn't question the environment; they question themselves. 'I must be unlovable,' 'My needs are wrong,' etc. These unconscious emotional conclusions form the blueprint of how they feel and function as adults. This is where inner child work becomes a powerful therapeutic tool—not as a metaphor, but as a somatic reality. This approach to healing focuses on forming a new relationship with your younger self, based on felt safety rather than logic.

In sessions, clients often find that when they meet their inner child with curiosity instead of shame, the body begins to soften. Beliefs like 'I am too much,' or 'I am a burden,' begin to unravel. The inner child's healing begins when we learn to decode the body's signals and reclaim the child within.

Priya sat across from me, her fingers tracing the outline of her throat as she described the sensation that had haunted her for years. 'It is like I am always bracing,' she said. 'But I don't know what for.' This was the work ahead. It was not just about understanding her pain but about teaching her body a new way to exist in the world.

7. Decoding the Body's Signals

We began with simple observation. I asked Priya to notice when the lump in her throat tightened. The goal was not to judge it or fix it, but simply to listen. Over the weeks, a pattern emerged. It worsened when she needed to set boundaries, when authority figures spoke over her, and when memories of that childhood betrayal surfaced. Her body was speaking in the only language it had left.

One session, as she described a conflict at work, her hand flew to her neck. 'There it is again,' she said. This time, instead of resisting, we got curious. 'What if this sensation isn't a problem to solve, but a message to understand?' I asked. Slowly, we connected the physical tension to its emotional counterpart: the stifled voice, the swallowed truths.

8. **Externalising the Pain**

Moving beyond the physical sensation, we gave form to her suffering. Priya drew the lump as a dark mass of tangled ropes. She gave it a voice: 'I am here to protect you. If you stay quiet, you will stay safe.' This externalisation allowed her to confront the protective function of her symptoms without shame.

We created rituals of release. She wrote letters to her twelve-year-old self and burned them. She practised pushing against my hands with her own while voicing boundaries she had never been allowed to set. We incorporated fantasy and imagery to access parts of her memory and emotion that words alone couldn't reach. With each act, her body learnt that expression didn't have to mean danger.

In therapy, fantasy can be accessed in a variety of ways, most notably through hypnotherapy. Using techniques like guided imagery, visualisation, meditation, mindfulness, and hypnosis, clients enter a relaxed, focused state in which they can safely explore inner experiences. The therapist invites the client to visualise specific scenarios—safe spaces, nurturing figures, or even their younger selves—to support emotional integration. This symbolic revisiting of painful moments, combined with new internal resources, allows for the reprocessing of past experiences. When practised repeatedly over time, this can promote deep nervous system regulation.

9. Reclaiming the Inner Child

The deepest work, though, came through visualisation. In guided sessions, Priya met her younger self in memory. She offered the child the words she had once needed: 'I believe you. It wasn't your fault.' At first, these moments brought violent shaking, as if her body was discharging decades of held energy. But over time, they became spaces of profound reconnection. One afternoon, Priya arrived with a change I could see before she even spoke. Her shoulders rested differently. 'The lump isn't gone,' she said. 'But it is quieter. Like it knows I am listening now.' This was the blueprint being rewritten. It was not happening through force but through faithful attention. A reconditioning of the mind and body towards safety. Several therapeutic tools support this work: breathwork, visualisations, affirmations, somatic tracking, and mindfulness meditation. These practices help shift the nervous system out of reactive survival states and into regulation. Over time, with repetition and emotional safety, the brain begins to form new neural associations. This is not about erasing the past but about creating new relational experiences inside the body and brain that gently counter the old survival programming.

10. It Is All in the Pause

Healing doesn't involve a juggernaut slamming through the walls one has built. More often, it begins with a quiet, unassuming pause. A pause that, when the body speaks through pain, tension, or illness, listens without judgement and simply asks: 'When did this first appear?' 'What was happening?' It is important to understand that healing isn't about erasing the past but about changing its relationship to the present. As Priya discovered, our bodies are not prisons of pain but living texts, always capable of new interpretations.

11. **Rituals of Repair**

    Ritual can serve as a powerful antidote to helplessness, transforming passive suffering into active ceremony. This was especially helpful in Priya's case, where intellectual insight alone couldn't ease the persistent tension in her throat. Her body had learnt its lessons in the old language—through touch, silence, and survival chemistry—so we spoke back in kind. So, when Priya burned her letters, the flames weren't just destroying words. They were rewriting her nervous system's expectations, i.e. what was once too dangerous to voice could now rise as smoke and ash. When she pushed against my hands to practice boundaries, her muscles weren't just moving; they were unlearning decades of 'stay small' with every resisted pound of force. Science calls this memory reconsolidation. It is the moment when old neural pathways destabilise and new experiences begin to overwrite fear's blueprint. But in my office, we called it teaching the body to unlearn.

12. **Final Letter to Her Younger Self**

    Priya hesitated before picking up the pen. 'What if I don't know what to say?' she asked.

    I handed her a sheet of paper and replied, 'The words already live in your body. We are just giving them a place to land.' This became our most powerful ritual. It did not erase her pain, but it honoured the child who had carried it for so long.

As Priya wrote to her twelve-year-old self, something remarkable happened. The sentences came haltingly at first, then in a flood:

- 'I am sorry no one believed you.'
- 'You were so brave to speak.'
- 'What happened wasn't your fault.'
- 'You don't have to protect them anymore.'

Her hands shook as she folded the letter. We stepped outside, and she lit a match, watching the flames transform decades of silence into smoke and ash. 'It feels like she can finally rest,' Priya whispered. And in that moment, her throat—that faithful, wounded sentinel—relaxed its grip.

13. The Role of Belief

Priya's journey shows what modern science now confirms that trauma changes our biology, but so does healing. Every time we tend to those wounded places with words, with witness, with deliberate care, we send new instructions to our cells. The throat learns it can open. The shoulders remember how to rest. The breath discovers its natural rhythm.

So, if childhood writes the body's first draft, belief edits the final copy. Unpacking those beliefs begins with understanding how thoughts become biology. This highlights the fact that healing and release aren't metaphors; they are a form of neural alchemy. This is the literal rewriting of cellular memory through attention and ritual.

Chapter 2

The Emotional Blueprint

'When we stop fearing the strange things we feel,
we begin to understand what they mean.'

Felt but Not Forgotten

The woman on my couch clutched her throat as if she were strangling herself. Medical scans showed nothing abnormal. She could eat, drink, and breathe without issue, but the sensation was real and relentless. 'It feels like I am being choked,' she whispered. 'Like there is a hand on my neck that no one else can see.'

She wasn't being strangled. Not now. But years ago, she had been—not by a pair of hands, but by something far more insidious: silence, rules, and the crushing weight of expectations no child should have to carry. Back then, speaking up wasn't safe. Expressing hurt wasn't allowed. So, her voice withdrew somewhere deep inside, buried under years of learnt restraint. And now, three decades later, her body still remembered what her mind had learnt to forget. Her neck muscles hadn't forgotten. They tightened around that unspoken fear, around words that had never been said aloud.

We often think of our emotions and feelings as fleeting experiences that come and go. But traumatic emotions, especially those from the past, don't simply disappear; they continue to live on in the body. The body remembers what it felt like to freeze when you wanted to run, to smile when you wanted to cry, to stay silent when you desperately needed to scream.

We often label these responses as dysfunction—symptoms, disorders, or maladaptations. But more often than not, they are not signs of a body gone wrong; they are signs of a body that adapted intelligently to overwhelming circumstances. What feels irrational today may have been the wisest survival strategy available at the time.

Think about it: if you were never safe to speak, it make perfect sense that your body might flinch at the idea of confrontation, or that your throat might tighten when you try to assert yourself. If affection was withheld or given conditionally, of course your nervous system might question intimacy now. These aren't flaws but survival codes written into the body. These can also be seen as messages left behind by your younger self.

The body, in this way, becomes a living record. It holds not just the events but also how we made sense of them, how we endured them, and what we had to put away in order to keep going. And unless those embodied emotions are seen, felt, and given space to be reprocessed, they don't simply fade. They echo . . . sometimes in pain, sometimes in tension, and sometimes in the strange and unexplainable symptoms that no scan can identify.

So, when we talk about healing, we are not only talking about the mind. We are talking about decoding the body's language. We are talking about re-establishing safety, both intellectually and physiologically. Because until the body feels safe, it cannot let go. It will hold on for dear life, not because something is malfunctioning but because it remains loyal to what once helped us survive.

This is why healing isn't just about rewiring thought patterns. Instead, it is about slowly, compassionately updating the body's memory of what it means to be alive. In that process, we don't just change behaviour, but we also begin to transform the very foundation of how safety, connection, and selfhood are felt.

The Blueprint Is Written Early

Every child is born with fundamental emotional needs: to feel seen, soothed, safe, and supported. We arrive in the world wired for connection, affection, comfort, and co-regulation. These early interactions form the emotional scaffolding upon which our sense of self is built. Whether our needs are consistently met or are neglected, distorted, or misunderstood, they shape the blueprint for how we relate to ourselves, to others, and to the world around us.

This shaping doesn't always come from obvious or traumatic events. More often, it unfolds in quiet, seemingly ordinary moments. These moments are so subtle that they often go unnoticed. A parent looks away when a child cries, not out of cruelty, but out of discomfort. A sibling mocks your joy, not from malice, but from mirroring what they have seen at home. A caregiver withdraws during conflict, and over time, silence becomes the language of tension. These experiences may not leave physical scars or dramatic memories, but they leave emotional imprints all the same.

Children are deeply perceptive but not yet equipped with the reasoning skills of adults. They don't think, 'My parent is overwhelmed' or 'My sibling is projecting their own pain.' Instead, they internalise these moments as truths about themselves—'I am too much,' 'My feelings don't matter,' or 'Love disappears when I am upset.' Over time, these interpretations become embedded in the psyche and eventually crystallise, subtly influencing how we show up in relationships and how we see ourselves for years to come.

Therefore, what starts as a response to specific moments—perhaps even moments forgotten—slowly becomes belief and belief becomes behaviour. And when that behaviour is repeated over and over, it hardens into personality, and we begin to mistake our adaptations for identity. We see this play out when a child who had to stay quiet to avoid upsetting the household grows up into an adult who apologises for simply taking up space. When a child's joy was never mirrored or acknowledged, they may become an adult who feels guilty for being happy. And when a child learns that expressing big emotions drives people away, they often become adults who hide their feelings in order to keep others close. What we often dismiss as 'just the way I am' is, in many cases, a collection of coping strategies that once kept us safe. These strategies get stored not just in our minds but in our bodies—in muscle tension, posture, tone of voice, and reflexive emotional responses. They form an emotional and physiological blueprint. It is a survival script written early and reinforced over time. And because this blueprint was developed so young, it often operates beneath conscious awareness. We don't remember choosing it. We just live it and find ourselves repeating dynamics in our lives, reacting in familiar ways, attracting similar patterns, unsure why we are stuck, until we begin to trace those patterns back to where they were first written.

Understanding this doesn't mean blaming our caregivers. Most were doing the best they could with what they knew. But recognising how our early environment shaped our emotional coding gives us a powerful opening: the opportunity to update the script. Because while the blueprint may have been written early, it is not permanent. We can learn to meet the needs that went unmet. We can give ourselves the affirmation, safety, and compassion we didn't receive then. And in doing so, we begin the work of rewriting the story through one gentle, conscious choice at a time.

Emotional Regulation: A Clinical View

When we think of trauma, we often imagine emotional wounds such as fear, grief, anger, or shame. But beneath these emotions lies a deeper imprint, one that resides in the body. Trauma, at its core, is not just something we feel; it is something our nervous system remembers. Long after an event has passed, the body may remain locked in a state of alert, unable to register that the danger is over. This is why many trauma survivors find themselves reacting with panic, numbness, or shutdown in seemingly ordinary moments. Their nervous systems are not dysfunctional. They are doing their best to protect.

To truly understand how belief systems, emotional memory, and therapeutic change work, we need to understand the nervous system. Specifically, how it responds to stress, how it becomes dysregulated, and most importantly, how it can be supported in returning to safety and balance.

A foundational concept in trauma-informed care is 'the window of tolerance,' introduced by Dr Dan Siegel. This refers to the range of arousal within which a person can function effectively. Inside this window, people can reflect, feel, and relate without becoming overwhelmed or shutting down. They remain present, emotionally responsive, and resilient. But trauma narrows this window, sometimes dramatically. The nervous system swings between hyperarousal (racing heart, panic, hypervigilance, etc.) and hypoarousal (numbness, fogginess, emotional disconnection, etc.). These are not malfunctions. They are the body's brilliant survival strategies, designed for short-term protection. But when they persist long after the threat has passed, they can interfere with daily life, relationships, and healing.

Traditional talk therapy, while valuable, often works through top-down processing, i.e., engaging the mind through language, reflection, and insight. But trauma resides in the body, and this is the reason why healing often requires a bottom-up approach that begins not with thoughts, but with the body. Breathwork, movement, somatic tracking, grounding techniques, and sensory awareness can slowly widen the window of tolerance, helping the nervous system feel safe enough to release its grip.

At the heart of this physiological recovery lies the vagus nerve—a key part of the parasympathetic nervous system, responsible for regulating the body's rest and digest functions. The vagus nerve connects the brainstem to almost every major organ, influencing heart rate, digestion, immunity, and emotional regulation. When the vagus nerve is well-regulated, the body becomes more resilient to stress and more capable of restoring balance after activation. When it is dysregulated, we see chronic inflammation, anxiety, gut issues, and difficulty connecting emotionally with others.

This is where many seemingly simple practices come into play. Humming, chanting, rhythmic breathing, singing, cold exposure, even making eye contact or speaking kindly—all of these can tone the vagus nerve. They are not superficial wellness trends; they are grounded in neuroscience. Each time we engage in these practices, we are sending a message to the body: You are safe now, and you can let go.

In trauma therapy, this work is not supplementary; it is foundational. Whether we use somatic experiencing, guided imagery, EMDR, or ritual-based practices, the aim is the same: to teach the body what safety feels like, again and again, until it becomes familiar. Only then can belief shift. Only then can emotional truth be reclaimed, not just as a story, but as a felt sense in the body. This is not a quick process. It requires patience, repetition, and compassion. But with time, the body begins to trust. The nervous system learns a new rhythm. And healing moves from something we know to something we live.

Case Study: Suppression as Symptom

Maya came to therapy because of chronic jaw pain. She had seen dentists, tried medication, and changed her diet, but nothing helped. Her pain was worse in the evenings and after meetings at work.

In her preliminary diagnosis, a recurring theme emerged: Maya often held back her opinions in professional settings, worried she'd be perceived as too aggressive. She had grown up in a family where speaking up invited criticism, and over time, had trained herself to remain agreeable and accommodating, even when it meant swallowing discomfort.

The jaw tension wasn't random. It was directly tied to the effort of restraint, of holding back emotion and words. The important point to note here is that our memories are not static archives; they evolve with our emotional states, often shaping how the body stores and reenacts past experiences.

Through somatic work and boundary-setting exercises, Maya began to notice when she was clenching and learnt how to interrupt the pattern early. She practised naming her needs in small, low-stakes situations, gradually building up to clearer communication at work. The pain didn't vanish overnight, but it eased as she grew more comfortable using her voice.

Case Study: Trust One's Gut

Raj was in his late thirties and had struggled with digestiv issues for nearly six years. He had been to specialists, tried elimination diets, probiotics, and medications. Nothing worked consistently. When we began working together, it became clear that his symptoms flared under pressure. They showed up before presentations, after disagreements with his partner, and whenever he took a break from work.

Raj had grown up under constant pressure to perform. Praise or approval came mostly when he achieved something. As a result, resting made him feel uneasy, even guilty. His body—especially his gut—responded strongly to anything that resembled failure, disconnection, or emotional vulnerability.

Therapy helped Raj connect these patterns. We worked on calming his nervous system, unpacking beliefs around rest and success, and slowly building a new internal narrative: that rest didn't have to be earned, and that failure didn't equate to rejection. Over time, his flare-ups reduced. And even when symptoms did arise, he no longer responded with fear.

Chapter 3
The Biology of Belief

'The body never lies. It whispers until we listen.'

Until now, we have looked at how emotional trauma imprints itself on the body. In this chapter, we will delve into the deep connection between mental states and physical well-being. It also introduces the concept of the science of belief, illustrating how thoughts and emotions can significantly influence the body's healing processes. Through a blend of scientific research, practical techniques, and compelling case studies, we will see how subconscious blocks, self-sabotaging tendencies, and emotional fragmentation can hinder well-being. Overcoming these internal barriers can result in powerful health transformations. The practices of self-reflection and meditation introduced in each chapter are designed to deepen your connection to your own mind and body.

You will also learn about the concept of locus of control, the importance of integrating various aspects of the self, and the healing power of imagination and personal narrative. The chapter also addresses the unique challenges faced by healers and underscores the importance of communal support in the healing journey. Overall, it offers a comprehensive approach to harnessing the mind's capacity for physical wellness, providing tools and strategies for achieving holistic health and well-being.

Healing the Body Through the Mind

The notion that our thoughts and emotions affect our physical health is no longer just intuitive; it is empirical. For much of its history, modern medicine treated the mind and body as two distinct domains. Illnesses were either psychological or physical, never both. But today, that binary view is dissolving. Lived experiences, body-based therapies, and a growing body of interdisciplinary research reveal just how profoundly our mental and emotional states shape the physical body and vice versa.

In therapeutic settings, people often seek help for anxiety, depression, trauma, or relational issues. Yet just as often, they arrive with symptoms that don't appear strictly psychological: chronic headaches, digestive troubles, unexplained fatigue, skin disorders, or autoimmune flares. These are not anomalies. More often than not, these physical complaints carry emotional narratives that the conscious mind may not yet have words for, but the body has already begun to express.

The human body is not a passive recipient of stress; it is a finely attuned barometer of it. Beliefs, especially those formed under prolonged emotional strain or during critical periods of development, shape the body's physiology. A nervous system trained to anticipate danger becomes overactive. This can manifest as insomnia, muscle tightness, shallow breathing, digestive irregularities, or hypersensitivity to sound or touch. These symptoms are often dismissed as 'just stress,' but they are actually the body's way of signalling unresolved emotion.

So, when shame takes root early in life, it doesn't just haunt thoughts; it curls the spine, collapses posture, and tightens the chest. When people describe themselves as 'feeling small' or 'wanting to disappear,' the body obliges. Shoulders hunch, breath shortens, and the entire system learns to dim itself down. Over time, this creates a loop: emotions shape posture, posture shapes breath, breath shapes perception, and the cycle continues. Thus, we can conclude that the story of the mind is, quite literally, written in the language of the body.

Yet what is profound about this interconnection is that it also holds the key to healing. When we work with the mind—by becoming aware of the beliefs we have internalised, the emotions we have exiled, the fears we keep feeding—we can begin to influence the body's state. And equally, when we work with the body through movement, breath, posture, and somatic awareness, we can shift the emotional patterns lodged in the psyche.

Healing, then, is not about fixing the mind or treating the body in isolation. It is about listening to how they speak to each other and allowing that dialogue to become conscious. Over time, this awareness becomes truly transformative. Panic begins to give way to presence, tension gradually softens into trust, and what once felt chronic starts to feel changeable. This is possible because the body not only remembers but it can also relearn.

Body Zones of Emotional Storage

Our bodies are not just vessels that carry us through life. In other words, they are living maps of our emotional history. And with time and through both research and therapeutic practice, a compelling truth has emerged: the body stores emotional experiences in specific, often predictable zones. This isn't mere metaphor but a felt reality for many, and an increasingly recognised phenomenon in somatic psychology.

Clients often come into therapy describing symptoms that defy clear medical explanation. A persistent ache in the lower back. A tight throat that seems to close up during confrontation. A chest that feels heavy despite normal test results. Eventually, patterns begin to reveal themselves. Individuals who carry a strong sense of duty or self-blame frequently report back pain as if the weight of responsibility is physically carried there. Those who suppress grief or unspoken sorrow may experience digestive troubles or a tightness in the throat that makes it hard to speak. Chronic headaches are often linked to the pressure of internal conflict, while clients with histories of abandonment or emotional neglect frequently describe constriction in the chest or difficulty breathing.

These patterns are not fixed rules or diagnostic tools. Everybody is unique. But they appear often enough, with remarkable consistency, to warrant attention and curiosity. They point us towards the possibility that symptoms are not just interruptions to our well-being; they are expressions of it.

In therapy, we don't begin by assigning meaning to a symptom. We begin by listening. A clenched stomach during confrontation may not just be about anxiety. It could be a residue of past fear, a body remembering how it once had to armour itself. A locked jaw may not just be a tension issue. It may be holding years of unspoken rage. Clients are often surprised to discover that their bodies remember things their conscious minds have long forgotten or never fully processed.

When clients begin to bring mindful awareness to these areas of the body—not with judgement, but with curiosity and compassion—something begins to shift. What once felt like a malfunction or weakness is now seen as adaptation, i.e., the body doing what it had to in order to survive or be accepted. We begin to realise that symptoms are not random. Tracking these sensations alongside emotional experiences opens up a deeper kind of dialogue. The ache in your shoulders during conflict might echo the bracing you once did as a child when arguments flared around you. The tension in your gut may stem from a time when you had to hold everything in in order to be strong, to not cause trouble, to survive.

This awareness doesn't necessarily erase the pain, but it transforms how we relate to it. Understanding where a pattern comes from creates context, and context gives us choice. We are no longer just trying to suppress symptoms or fix the body. We are learning to interpret its signals, to speak its language, and to respond with care instead of fear. In doing so, we shift from seeing the body as a battleground to honouring it as a messenger that has always been on our side, asking to be heard.

Psychoneuroimmunology: The Mind-Body Interaction

Psychoneuroimmunology (PNI) is the study of how mental processes influence the nervous and immune systems. Put simply, it highlights how profoundly emotional states can impact physical health. For instance, chronic stress—a mentally taxing condition—has been shown to suppress immune function, making the body more vulnerable to illness. Similarly, negative emotions and limiting beliefs can weaken the immune system and pave the way for disease. Conversely, positive mental states—such as hope, joy, or optimism—can enhance immune performance. These effects are largely mediated by the neuroendocrine system, which regulates interactions between the brain, hormones, and immune response.

When stress becomes chronic, the body secretes increased levels of cortisol, which is a hormone that, in excess, impairs immune function. On the other hand, positive emotions have been shown to increase levels of immunoglobulins and natural killer cells, both of which are essential to defending the body against pathogens.

This dynamic relationship between belief and biology is mediated through interconnected systems—the brain, endocrine system, and immune system—with the brain, particularly the hypothalamus, playing a central role. The hypothalamus regulates both the autonomic and endocrine systems. In response to stress, it triggers the release of cortisol and adrenaline. Yet, in states of calm or connection, it can stimulate the production of oxytocin—often referred to as the trust and love hormone—which actively counters the effects of stress and supports immune function.

In essence, even the expectation of relief or healing can trigger neurochemical changes that promote well-being. When belief is positively directed, it functions as a powerful biological agent of change by initiating real, measurable changes in the body and mind. This highlights the profound connection between perception, belief, and physiology, reminding us that the mind's influence on health is not just psychological but deeply physical as well.

Neuroplasticity

Neuroplasticity refers to the brain's remarkable ability to reorganise its structure and function in response to life experiences, emotional states, and belief systems. Once believed to be relatively fixed after childhood, the brain is now understood to remain adaptable throughout life—a point made powerfully in Norman Doidge's *The Brain That Changes Itself*. This adaptability plays a key role not only in learning and memory but also in emotional healing and psychological growth.

Neuroscientists have found that the brain can rewire itself based on experience, which has profound implications for mental health. For instance, someone who has lived in chronic fear may have neural pathways that are conditioned to anticipate threat. But with time, emotional safety, and consistent therapeutic practices—such as mindfulness, breathwork, or talk therapy—new pathways can be formed. These alternative circuits support calm, curiosity, and trust, gradually replacing old patterns of fear, shame, or self-criticism.

This flexibility of the brain explains why healing is not just psychological but also physiological. Therapeutic relationships that offer presence, attunement, and care can initiate changes in the brain. People often report physical improvements—reduced chronic pain, digestive relief, or better sleep—not only because of techniques used in therapy but because they feel heard, held, and understood. Emotional states like happiness and safety trigger the release of neurochemicals such as endorphins, which function as the body's natural painkillers, often rivalling pharmaceutical effects.

Even in conditions like depression, anxiety, or Parkinson's disease, patients have shown measurable improvement simply through the belief that they are getting better. Such findings reveal a powerful truth: the mind, when positively engaged, becomes a catalyst for healing and sometimes as significant as medical intervention itself.

Thus, we can conclude that pain, trauma, and emotional distress are not imagined, but they are also not fixed. They are expressions of how the mind and body interact, and thanks to neuroplasticity, what has been conditioned can also be deconditioned. The story of the mind is written in the language of the body, and that story can, with care and effort, be rewritten.

Recurring Themes in Body-Belief Research

While individual experiences vary greatly, there is a striking consistency in the psychological undercurrents that shape how the body responds to belief. Across different cultures, socioeconomic backgrounds, and clinical presentations, certain themes keep resurfacing, pointing not only to the profound link between the psyche and the soma but also to the shared human longing for meaning, coherence, and safety.

One of the most prominent themes that emerges is the enduring impact of early life experiences. Childhood environments—particularly those marked by emotional neglect, inconsistency, or trauma—can give rise to core beliefs that settle deep within the nervous system. Over time, these beliefs, often unconscious, begin to script the body's responses to life. For example, a child who learnt that love is conditional may grow into an adult whose body braces under even minor interpersonal conflict. The posture stiffens and the breath shortens, not because there is actual danger, but because the body remembers what the mind cannot fully recall.

Cultural narratives also shape these internalised patterns. In some communities, emotional expression is discouraged, seen as weak or shameful. In others, stoicism is valorised while vulnerability is pathologised. Clients internalise these cultural messages, leading to embodied dissonance: emotions arise naturally, but their expression is blocked or distorted. Over time, this emotional repression can take a physical toll, resulting in headaches, gastrointestinal distress, or chronic fatigue. As such, belief and biology become entangled in ways that medical science alone cannot fully explain. This disconnect between lived experience and clinical interpretation often leaves individuals feeling unseen.

Moreover, many clients interviewed in long-form case studies shared a common frustration: their physical symptoms had been repeatedly dismissed by medical professionals because test results showed 'nothing wrong.' Yet in therapeutic spaces where symptoms were held with curiosity instead of suspicion, a different truth emerged. Their pain was not imaginary; it was intelligent. The body, having no words, had simply found other ways to speak.

These stories reinforce a critical distinction that healing does not necessarily mean replacing wrong beliefs with right ones. Rather, it involves contextualising those beliefs, i.e., understanding when, how, and why they formed. When clients begin to see their physiological responses not as malfunctions but as once-adaptive survival strategies, the grip of shame often loosens. In its place, a wave of clarity may arise. For some, this clarity brings grief, a mourning for the years spent feeling broken or misunderstood. But for many, it also brings self-compassion and a renewed sense of agency.

Ultimately, we can see how belief shapes biology, but it's important to remember that the process isn't one-way. The body is not static; it learns, adapts, and responds to new experiences. With time, safety, and fresh insight, the physiological responses that once served to protect can be softened, even rewired. When the internal world becomes safer than the one that birthed the original belief, the body no longer needs to carry the same burden. This is the heart of embodied healing, not the erasure of pain but the re-authoring of its meaning.

Practical Implications

The effects of the biology of belief on the body and overall health have significant practical implications in the fields of medicine and personal well-being. This clearly suggests that improving mental health should not be pursued solely for the sake of achieving a better state of mind, as it can also result in tangible benefits for physical health. Various mind-body interventions, such as meditation, mindfulness, and psychological therapies, are useful in shifting limiting beliefs to create more favourable health outcomes.

The goal of therapy and healing is ultimately to help individuals find balance by integrating different aspects of themselves, including the mental and physical selves. Ideally, the ability to maintain a mental and physical balance should come naturally to most people. Yet, over time, the skill of knowing thyself often becomes clouded and neglected in favour of a fast-paced lifestyle shaped by the demands and constant motion of modern life. While this pace is necessary to keep up with societal expectations, it is also deeply damaging to one's physiological and psychological health. Without it, one may fall behind, and with it, stress becomes a constant companion. This ongoing stress often manifests physically—as headaches, migraines, insomnia, strain injuries, muscular disorders, and back pain—as well as psychologically, in the form of cognitive disturbances like restlessness, poor focus, anxiety, depression, and even addiction. Prolonged exposure to stress also contributes to more serious conditions such as immune disorders, hypertension, heart disease, and cancer.

In the end, healing is not about escape but return to the body, to the breath, and to the beliefs that quietly shape the way we feel and function. It is through this return that change becomes possible.

In the following sections, we will explore how the mind and body can be brought into greater harmony through simple yet powerful practices like guided meditation. We will also examine a case study that illustrates how individuals who initially seek therapy for physical issues often uncover deeper psychological roots and how addressing these can lead to profound physical relief.

Guided Meditation: Healing and Balancing Body and Mind

In a world that constantly pulls us outward, guided meditation offers a chance to reconnect with ourselves in a deeper way. It creates a safe, intentional space where the body can soften and the mind can settle, allowing healing to begin from within.

In the guided meditation that follows, each step is designed to gently guide you toward healing and restoring balance between body and mind.

1. **Preparation**

   Find a quiet, calm space where you will not be disturbed for the next 15-20 minutes. Settle into a comfortable position—either sitting or lying down—and follow the steps below after closing your eyes.

2. **Take a Seat or Recline**

   Settle into a sitting or reclining position, whichever feels most comfortable. Let your body relax and ease into stillness. When you feel ready, gently close your eyes and begin to breathe deeply in through your nose and out through your mouth. With every exhalation, release any tension you may be holding on to, allowing yourself to relax even more deeply.

3. **Body Scan**

   Once your breath has settled, bring your awareness to your body and begin a gentle mental scan from head to toe or from toe to head, whichever feels natural. Gradually move your attention across every part of your body, noticing any areas of tension or discomfort. As you identify those areas, visualise yourself breathing into them. With each inhalation, imagine your breath reaching deep into those tissues and muscles; with each exhalation, visualise the tension loosening and those areas softening and relaxing.

4. **Visualisation**

   Now, begin to picture a warm, healing light entering your body with every breath in. Let this light take the form of a vivid, golden glow, full of life-giving energy. With each inhalation, imagine this golden light spreading through your entire body, enveloping every cell, muscle, and organ. Feel this light as peaceful, restorative energy bringing renewal to your system. With every breath out, imagine releasing pain, stress, or sickness. Picture these leaving your body as heavy, dark clouds dissolving into the atmosphere. Continue this cycle—breathing in healing light, breathing out heaviness and stagnation—until you feel your body becoming lighter, more open, and increasingly energised.

5. **Affirmations**

   As you breathe and visualise the healing light, support the process further by mentally repeating affirmations that resonate with you. For example:

   - 'My body is on the path to recovery.'
   - 'I am fully healthy.'
   - 'My entire being is active and healthy at the cellular level.'
   - 'I exist in a harmonious mind-body-soul relationship.'

Repeat these affirmations with heartfelt intention and positive energy, fully connecting with the meaning behind each statement. Let them settle into your consciousness and become a part of your being. Such affirmations can powerfully support the healing of your entire system.

6. **Integration and Closing**

   After spending a few minutes in visualisation and affirmations, gently bring your awareness back to your breath. Breathe deeply and settle into the here and now. Acknowledge the connection between your mind and body and the healing process you have set in motion. When you feel ready, slowly return your attention to your surroundings. You may begin to notice the movement of your fingers and toes and become aware of your breath again. When you are ready, open your eyes and come back feeling refreshed, renewed, and deeply connected to your body and mind.

Case Study: Stress and Health

Karan presented a range of physical symptoms, including irritable bowel syndrome (IBS), abdominal pain, breathing difficulties, allergies, heel pain, headaches, and a history of kidney stones. In addition, he reported suffering from insomnia, chronic fatigue, anxiety, low motivation, frustration, and depressive feelings.

Many of Karan's physical issues were linked to unhealthy lifestyle choices made during his youth, including both active and passive smoking, and excessive consumption of energy drinks. At the time of seeking therapy, most conventional treatments had shown limited effectiveness, and medical evaluations had revealed no underlying physical cause. The absence of a clear diagnosis only compounded his stress and depression.

Moreover, Karan's case history revealed a lack of strong emotional bonds within the family, contributing to a persistent sense of loneliness and a limited social network. The absence of emotional connection and support from a young age often led to feelings of rejection and isolation that persisted into adulthood.

The primary goal of therapy for Karan was to release both emotional and physical pain. A central part of this work involved externalising the pain, i.e., engaging with it as a separate entity outside the self. This process combined gestalt and psychodrama techniques such as externalisation, projection, roleplay, and the empty chair technique. By addressing pain from an externalised, objective standpoint, clients often gained clarity and insight into their emotional burdens. Separating their identity from the pain allowed them to begin understanding the roots of their suffering more effectively.

During one session, Karan recalled feeling overwhelmed by academic and work pressures in his youth, stating that his unhealthy coping habits originated during this period. These anxieties, which offered momentary relief at the time, gradually caused long-term harm to both body and mind. He was encouraged to externalise each emotion associated with this period and work through them individually. This helped him recognise how, somewhere along the way, he began valuing his body less, prioritising academic and career success instead. Reclaiming a sense of self-love and reconnecting with his body as a valuable, worthy part of his life became a crucial aspect of Karan's healing.

Later in the session, Karan was guided through relaxation and imagery-based techniques to help manage stress more effectively. He described feeling dazed yet refreshed afterwards and noted a marked reduction in physical pain. He was invited to continue therapy to gradually release the cumulative stress that had taken a toll on his body. Although Karan had already given up the unhealthy habits of his past, he now expressed a renewed commitment to investing in his health and fitness. As a result, self-care became a cornerstone of his recovery process.

It is vitally important to recognise the deep interconnection between mental and physical health. The two are in constant dialogue, and sustained wellness depends on achieving a balance between mind and body. Self-love and self-care—often overlooked in conventional medical and therapeutic settings—are finally receiving the attention they deserve, with visible benefits when integrated into the healing process.

Chapter 4
Locus of Control

'Every time you reclaim your choice, you reclaim a piece of yourself.'

This chapter can greatly support readers on their life journey by helping them recognise just how much influence they hold over their own lives. It addresses an individual's belief about the degree to which they control the events that affect them. For instance, individuals who engage in constant people-pleasing often operate with an external locus of control. For such people, life can feel particularly difficult because there is always someone around them who remains unhappy, no matter how much they do.

By understanding and mastering their own locus of control, readers can develop a stronger sense of personal agency and enhance their overall well-being. The purpose of this chapter is to raise awareness about how one's life events are being guided. From there, the choice to change or to continue living in the same way rests entirely in their hands, through the power of free will. Recognising where control truly lies is the first step towards reclaiming personal power. To better understand this dynamic, let's explore the concept of the locus of control in more detail.

Understanding Locus of Control

The locus of control refers to a person's beliefs around control and personal power. An internal locus of control reflects the belief that one has the ability to shape their own life and circumstances. In contrast, an external locus of control involves believing that life is directed by outside forces such as government, fate, nature, or a deity.

One of the greatest barriers to healing is the belief that one lacks the power to create change. An external locus of control can strip an individual of their sense of agency and lead to avoidance of personal responsibility. It may also result in feelings of helplessness, frustration, anger, resentment, and a lack of trust, both in others and in oneself. This belief system can lead people to habitually blame others for their life experiences, thereby reinforcing a victim mindset. In Jungian archetypes, the victim is someone who sees themselves as repeatedly wronged and absolves themselves of all responsibility, often reinforced by the sympathy or pity they receive from others. This often results in a sense of being stuck and unable to change one's circumstances. In such situations, what's typically needed is a shift in perspective—one that empowers the individual to see themselves as the author of their own life, capable of healing and shaping the reality they seek. In such situations, what is typically needed is a shift in perspective that empowers the individual to see themselves as the author of their own life, capable of healing and shaping the reality they seek.

Cultivating an internal locus of control is not about denying real-world limitations or injustices, but about reclaiming the power to respond consciously, rather than reactively. When individuals begin to realise that they can choose their thoughts, actions, and responses—even in the face of difficulty—they begin to reclaim a profound sense of agency. This shift lays the foundation for true psychological and physiological healing.

Self-Sabotage and the Manifestation of Fear

Self-sabotage is a crucial aspect to consider as it often reflects a pattern of unconsciously obstructing one's own growth. This may take the form of mental blocks—such as unconscious beliefs or thoughts that hinder progress—or physical blocks, including recurring habits or behavioural patterns that derail movement towards personal goals.

A common trait among individuals who self-sabotage is an external locus of control, i.e., a belief that external forces dictate their actions and destiny. These individuals often experience a sense of helplessness when it comes to taking charge of their own lives or assuming responsibility for their outcomes. Key focus areas in therapeutic work with such clients include confidence and self-esteem, underlying insecurities, lack of independence, depressive symptoms (especially those involving hopelessness and helplessness), and a deep-seated belief that they are incapable of changing their reality.

What makes self-sabotage particularly insidious is that it often masquerades as protection, such as avoiding risk, staying safe, or managing expectations. But beneath this protective facade lies fear of failure, fear of success, or fear of stepping into an unfamiliar identity. In therapy, the work involves gently bringing these fears to the surface, understanding their origins, and cultivating inner safety so that growth no longer feels like a threat. Helping individuals reconnect with their own agency and reframe challenges as opportunities is central to breaking the cycle of self-sabotage.

Steps to Shift Locus of Control

Shifting from an external to an internal locus of control is a gradual, intentional process that begins with self-awareness and is strengthened through practical action. The steps below offer concrete strategies to help you reclaim a sense of agency, build confidence in your ability to influence outcomes, and move towards a more empowered way of living.

1. **Assess Your Locus of Control**

   The first step in shifting your perception of control is determining whether your current locus of control is internal or external. Reflect on your thoughts and feelings and ask yourself who you believe is truly responsible for what happens in your life. When you hear about someone's success, do you think, 'That was all them,' or do you believe, 'They were just lucky,' or 'It was their circumstances'? Similarly, when you succeed, do you credit your effort or external factors? Gaining awareness of how you attribute control will help you take the first step towards meaningful change.

2. **Engage in Empowerment Exercises**

   Consciously choose to engage in exercises and activities that help you build a sense of control. Identify short-term, achievable goals that gradually shift your perception from external to internal control and build your confidence along the way. For example, instead of making a broad statement like, 'I want to get fit,' break it down to 'I will work out three times a week.' Each time you achieve that small goal, acknowledge the effort you put in and the outcome you created. This helps build the belief that your actions lead to results and that you have the ability to create positive change.

3. **Support Yourself with Cognitive-Behavioural Therapy**

   If you consistently feel like you have little or no control over your life, this can impact your overall well-being. In such cases, seeking the support of a therapist may be helpful. Cognitive behavioural therapy (CBT) is especially effective in helping individuals shift towards an internal locus of control. CBT focuses on identifying and changing dysfunctional thought patterns and behaviours, and on strengthening personal coping strategies. Through this work, you begin to realise how much influence you truly have over your mental health and the direction of your life.

Guided Meditation: Internalising Control

The following guided meditation is designed to help internalise your sense of control, grounding your power within rather than placing it outside of yourself. It offers a gentle yet powerful way to reconnect with your inner agency, especially when life feels uncertain or overwhelming. By tapping into visualisation, breath, and intention, this practice supports the deep belief that you can influence your reality. Let it serve as a reminder that the ability to steer your life lies not in external circumstances, but in the choices you make moment to moment.

1. **Preparation**

   Choose a quiet, undisturbed space where you can relax for the next 20–30 minutes. Find a comfortable position—either sitting or lying down—and gently close your eyes.

2. **Unwind and Relax**

   Get into a cosy position, close your eyes, and begin to breathe slowly and deeply. Inhale through your nose, hold the breath for a moment, and then exhale fully through your mouth. With each breath, allow your body to relax more deeply than before. Feel the tension leaving your muscles. Let your mind begin to settle into stillness.

3. **Take Control of Your Life**

   Now, imagine your life as a car, and you are in the driver's seat. Your hands are on the steering wheel, firm and steady. Visualise yourself confidently steering this car, guiding it in the direction you choose. Let this image remind you that you are in control. The direction your life takes is shaped by the choices you make.

4. **Empowerment through Constructive Self-Affirmations**

   As you hold this steering wheel, affirm your power to yourself. Let these words rise from within and echo through your being:

   - 'I am in charge of my life.'
   - 'I take steps that serve my highest good.'
   - 'I am capable and empowered.'
   - 'I take action, and it leads to positive outcomes.'

   Repeat these affirmations a few times. With each repetition, notice how your sense of confidence and inner control grows stronger.

5. **Future Visualisation**

Now, visualise yourself moving through life with clarity and ease. Picture yourself handling challenges with strength and purpose. Imagine scenarios where you step up and take the lead, whether that is restoring your health, reaching personal milestones, or overcoming obstacles. See yourself thriving, achieving, and living fully.

As you witness these images, feel the power within you. Recognise that you are the architect of your reality through your intentions, choices, and actions.

6. **Closing**

Take a few deep, steady breaths. Feel a renewed sense of control and empowerment spreading through you. Let this feeling anchor itself in your body and mind. When you are ready, begin to bring your awareness back to the room. Gently wiggle your fingers and toes. When you feel ready, open your eyes, carrying with you a deep sense of inner strength and the knowledge that you are capable of steering your life in the direction you choose.

Case Study: Constraints and the Journey into Freedom

Nikhil held a deep belief in external forces determining fate and felt powerless to change the course of his life. He presented with intense fear and anxiety related to the unknown, failure, and death, and described feeling immobilised and stuck in a loop of inaction. Nikhil struggled with forming close connections and found it difficult to stay emotionally present in existing relationships. At the same time, he placed high importance on achieving career success, financial stability, and discovering his life's purpose.

Nikhil frequently mentioned his mother, described as a highly anxious person. He was also dealing with paranoia, hallucinations, disrupted sleep, chronic fatigue, and challenges with maintaining personal hygiene. Interestingly, while he identified his mother as a constraint, he also viewed her as his primary support system. This contradiction revealed the complexity of his emotional attachment.

In understanding constraints and the locus of control, it was essential to explore attachment dynamics and how early relationships shaped adult interactions. Anxious parenting and attachment patterns in early childhood were often linked to similar patterns of anxiety and insecurity in adulthood. These dynamics impacted a person's ability to explore freely, develop healthy relationships, and reach their full potential. Nikhil acknowledged experiencing difficulty in all of these areas and attributed much of it to the overarching feeling of being constrained.

He also discussed his parents' troubled marriage and how his determination to never become like them may have, paradoxically, contributed to similar issues within his own marriage. This pointed to the presence of subconscious oaths or internal vows—decisions made in response to past pain—which, when left unchecked, could end up creating the very circumstances they were intended to avoid. This was a classic example of a self-fulfilling prophecy, where fear of a particular outcome caused behaviours that ultimately brought that outcome to life.

Given Nikhil's anxious tendencies—especially his habit of overthinking and engaging in repetitive thought loops—conventional talk therapy proved difficult. Instead, alternative methods such as grounding meditations and hypnotherapy were introduced. These approaches helped him remain mindful, relaxed, and more present. Nikhil also began journaling regularly to track and process his thoughts and feelings.

As sessions progressed to cover financial and career aspirations, Nikhil shared a strong desire to create something meaningful. He expressed that if more people understood him, he would be able to fulfil this goal, which once again highlighted his reliance on external validation and approval. Initially, he had expressed fear around expansion and the unknown; later, however, he began speaking with enthusiasm about growth and creation. Nikhil acknowledged that these changes were the result of therapeutic work that allowed him to explore and confront his fears.

Further discussion revealed that while Nikhil had always had great ideas and aspirations, he rarely received the encouragement needed to bring these ideas to life. In particular, his mother appeared to have been a significant source of anxiety and was unable to support his journey towards self-actualisation and creative expression. This lack of support tied into Nikhil's feelings of inadequacy, unimportance, and helplessness in influencing his own reality. An anxious attachment style, as discussed earlier, could severely hinder one's ability to develop a strong sense of self, trust their own instincts, and move forward with clarity and confidence.

When asked to engage in a future progression exercise—envisioning his goals manifesting into reality—Nikhil found the visualisation difficult. Once again, the sense of being constrained arose. He expressed a strong aversion to doing work he didn't enjoy or feel was necessary and instead spoke of a desire to engage in something he loved, ideally helping others through it. When prompted to imagine a life without constraints, Nikhil described it as a life of accomplishment but quickly added that such a state would only be temporary, as new constraints would inevitably arise. He also mentioned that such a life might feel lonely.

As discussed earlier, the abandoned or orphaned inner child often carries deep feelings of rejection and loneliness, stemming from an absence of emotional support during childhood. For Nikhil, the idea of a constraint-free life was difficult to imagine, not only because of its unfamiliarity, but also because he equated emotional bonds with restriction. In other words, Nikhil struggled to separate meaningful relationships from the experience of being emotionally constrained.

To support a shift from constraint to empowerment, Nikhil was guided through a visualisation exercise. He was asked to return to childhood memories and begin to externalise them through projection, speaking from his younger self to the family members who contributed to his anxious tendencies. When asked where his power lay, Nikhil responded: 'In the rewiring of the brain.' This revealed an important insight: he recognised that change began with a shift in perspective. However, when it came time to actively verbalise what he wanted to change, Nikhil retreated once again into a sense of powerlessness. He described feeling as if he were floating in space, unanchored and incapable of changing the weight of the past.

Nikhil frequently expressed a wish to create, contribute, and help others, but this dream was overshadowed by fear . . . fear of failure and fear of the responsibility that would come with actually succeeding. In many ways, remaining in the space of constraints offered a kind of safety, as it postponed the need to build emotional resilience or confront difficult truths. It was easier for Nikhil to remain suspended in the metaphorical 'outer space' than to ground himself in reality, where real-world challenges and healing had to take place.

After the visualisation, a discussion was held around the themes of personal responsibility, the desire to escape, and the difference between being empowered and actively reclaiming one's own power. Nikhil had been unable to change his life as a child and, as an adult, now dreamt of changing the world. His childhood experience of anxious parenting and lack of support contributed heavily to his current inner world, and therapy became the space in which these patterns were unlearnt. In shedding these inherited constraints, Nikhil began to make space for his authentic goals and the possibility of achieving them.

By the end of therapy, Nikhil had begun exploring new activities and working towards personal goals and dreams. He chose to enter the healing profession, aligning with his desire to help others. He had also begun to ground himself more firmly in the present moment and had learnt to live with greater awareness and presence. Most significantly, Nikhil had undergone a key internal shift: he gave himself permission to live his own life and make decisions for himself. This move towards a more internal locus of control brought about meaningful transformation, both in how he thought and how he lived.

Case Study: Restraints and Self-Actualisation

Meera presented with feelings of being held back from her true potential. She felt stuck, unable to reach larger goals, and experienced a sense of internal restraint. Meera acknowledged that this had caused her considerable stress. She described herself as highly intelligent but felt she had been unlucky in life. While she struggled academically when she was younger, she gradually improved. Despite expressing self-appreciation, Meera also demonstrated harsh self-judgement. She believed success was a mix of luck and hard work, yet viewed hard work primarily as a mental effort and often judged herself for not doing enough. She described herself as perfectionistic and admitted to compulsive tendencies, including holding grudges or seeking revenge. Meera operated with an external locus of control. While she believed her actions had power—as seen in her assertion that her then-current success was a form of revenge against doubters—nearly all of her decisions were rooted in reactions to what others had done or said to her. Once again, subconscious vows were evident in this case, i.e., a deep-seated drive to prove others wrong, rather than to pursue what she genuinely desired. Meera had unknowingly built a life focused not on personal goals, but on defying others' expectations. She had never aimed for success on her own terms; she had only chased the fulfilment of proving others wrong. Healing for Meera lay in learning to let go of these reactive patterns and beginning to live for herself. By releasing the vows made in opposition to others, she created space to discover and pursue her true dreams and ultimately, to manifest a reality aligned with her authentic self.

Chapter 5

Clinical Approaches to Belief Work

'Even the most implausible beliefs make perfect sense inside the system that created them.'

When Belief Meets Therapy

In therapeutic work, we often encounter clients whose lived experiences include visions, voices, premonitions, curses, karmic fears, ancestral communication, and spirit visitations. These beliefs may at first appear fantastical or irrational, especially when viewed through a strictly clinical lens. But in many cases, they are not signs of delusion or dysfunction. Instead, they serve as deeply meaningful symbolic systems formed through personal history, shaped by cultural narratives, and reinforced by the nervous system's attempt to interpret and survive overwhelming events.

These experiences are often dismissed too quickly in mainstream settings, labelled as 'symptoms' to be corrected rather than messages to be understood. But in therapy, particularly when working through trauma, the symbolic holds weight. The language of metaphor, imagery, and sensation is often the only language the body has when words fall short. A vision or visitation may not be literally true, but that doesn't make it untrue. It reflects something emotionally accurate: a story the psyche needed to tell when no other story could be told safely.

Frameworks like cognitive behavioural therapy (CBT) help bring structure to this process. They uncover the hidden narratives beneath symptoms. For example, a persistent stomach ache becomes 'I can't digest what I am being told,' while a recurring rash becomes 'I need space from contact.' But when the symptom is not just physical but symbolic or spiritual, belief work requires a different kind of gentleness. A client who believes they are cursed may not benefit from being told it isn't real. What they often need instead is safety and a space where that belief can be unpacked, not disproven. Dismissing these narratives outright can reinforce shame or abandonment. Understanding them, however, can open a door to healing.

As discussed earlier, beliefs are not just thoughts; they are somatic memories. They are the body's way of holding what the mind couldn't. Many clients carry beliefs not as chosen ideologies, but as adaptive truths born of experience. A child who was repeatedly betrayed may grow into an adult who believes the world is unsafe or that punishment is inevitable. These beliefs can take spiritual form, such as visions of retribution, voices of warning, or ancestral figures that echo the lessons of trauma.

Clinical language can help us navigate these experiences, offering clarity and tools. But it can also limit us. The way we name things determines how we approach them. A diagnosis might offer relief and explanation, but it can also become a fixed identity, overshadowing the full story. Especially when it comes to beliefs shaped by trauma, culture, or symbolic meaning, rigid definitions can stifle rather than support.

In this chapter, we explore the nuanced terrain where belief, trauma, and physiology intersect with modern diagnostic systems. The goal is not to validate every belief as truth, nor to erase them under the weight of scientific language. Rather, we aim to reclaim these narratives—to understand how they protect, guide, and express—and to support healing not through dismissal, but through deep listening. Sometimes, the most irrational-seeming belief is the most honest expression of pain. And sometimes, that expression is the first step towards wholeness.

The Clinical Frame: Understanding Mental Disorders

Before we can explore the symbolic and emotional dimensions of belief, it is important to understand how mainstream psychology and psychiatry define and approach certain mental health conditions, particularly those that involve shifts in perception, thought, and behaviour. Within the clinical frame, disorders like schizophrenia, bipolar disorder, and psychotic disorders are understood primarily in terms of neurochemical imbalance, cognitive distortion, and functional impairment. While this medical model provides structure and language to address suffering, it often struggles to account for the subjective, relational, and even spiritual meaning people assign to their experiences.

Let's briefly review the core features of these diagnoses:

- Schizophrenia is considered a severe and chronic psychiatric condition, typically emerging in early adulthood. It is marked by hallucinations (auditory or visual), delusions (fixed, false beliefs), disorganised speech or behaviour, and emotional withdrawal or flat affect. These symptoms can lead to significant difficulty in daily functioning. Standard treatment involves antipsychotic medication and psychosocial interventions designed to reduce distress and improve coping.

- Bipolar disorder involves mood instability characterised by episodes of mania and depression. Manic phases may include elevated mood, grandiosity, decreased need for sleep, and impulsive or risky behaviour. Depressive episodes are marked by hopelessness, lethargy, and social withdrawal. The rapid shifts between these states can be disorienting, not only for the individual but also for those around them, often leading to stigma or misinterpretation.
- Psychosis is not a standalone diagnosis but a symptom cluster that involves a break from shared reality, often through hallucinations, delusions, or disorganised thinking. Psychotic symptoms can occur in schizophrenia and bipolar disorder, but also in trauma-related conditions such as PTSD, or even in short-term states triggered by grief, sleep deprivation, or substance use.

While these diagnostic categories are important for structuring care and guiding interventions, they don't always capture the rich inner world of the person experiencing them. A hallucination may not simply be a malfunction of the brain; it could also be a metaphor, a memory, or an attempt by the psyche to make meaning of chaos. A manic episode might, in some cases, be a surge of suppressed creativity or emotion long denied. This doesn't mean we disregard clinical realities, but rather, we complement them with compassion, curiosity, and context.

By holding both the clinical and symbolic lenses, we can begin to ask not only 'What is wrong with you?' but also 'What happened to you and how has your system adapted to survive it?' In doing so, we lay the groundwork for care that honours both the biology and the biography of the person in front of us.

Reframing Disorders as Trauma Responses

We often enter the world of mental health through labels and terms such as schizophrenia, bipolar disorder, or psychosis that promise clarity and direction. These diagnoses, rooted in decades of clinical research, offer a structure for understanding distress. Yet when we look closely—not just through a clinical lens, but through the eyes of lived experience—these disorders begin to reveal something deeper: they are not malfunctions, but messages. Not fixed pathologies, but nervous systems in survival mode, shaped by histories of fear, neglect, and pain. To truly understand what lies beneath these conditions, we need to widen the lens and consider the body's role in holding memory and meaning.

A trauma-informed perspective provides a more comprehensive and compassionate framework for understanding these conditions. Rather than rushing to correct or suppress what appears broken, this lens invites us to listen, to slow down, and to understand that beneath every extreme state is a story the body remembers when the mind cannot. This shift allows us to move from pathologising to contextualising, from diagnosing to decoding.

In other words, it recognises that symptoms often emerge as adaptations, which were once necessary for survival, now misfiring in safer contexts. Instead of simply medicating away the symptoms, we begin to explore their purpose, their timing, and their voice. Such an approach doesn't deny biology; it expands it, honouring the intricate dance between brain chemistry and lived experience. In doing so, we offer the individual more than treatment. We offer dignity, a chance to be seen not as a diagnosis, but as a human being with a story that makes sense.

Rethinking Hallucinations and Delusions

In therapeutic practice, I have worked with clients who hear voices that are not symbolic, but vividly real. Often, they are the voices of abusive caregivers, echoing years after the trauma occurred. These are not simply hallucinations in the pathological sense. They are the nervous system's living memories, auditory imprints of terror, shame, or helplessness that were never processed or validated.

Seen this way, delusions and hallucinations may not be signs of madness but creative attempts at survival. The belief 'I am chosen' may protect a person from the unbearable core belief 'I am powerless.' The fear of being watched may mirror the hypervigilance born in unsafe homes. What appears irrational often follows a deep, internal logic that deserves respect.

1. **Bipolar States as Nervous System Extremes**

   The pendulum swing of mania and depression is often reduced to chemical imbalance. But for many clients, these states are intimately tied to how their nervous systems learnt to cope with instability. Put simply, Mania may have once been a lifeline, a way to feel in control, capable, or even euphoric in the face of chaos. In contrast, depression can be the body's intelligent shutdown, a retreat into numbness when everything feels too much.

   Therefore, we need to view these fluctuations not as dysfunction, but as natural, adaptive rhythms. This implies that healing doesn't mean flattening the highs and lows, but helping the person find regulation, safety, and choice within them.

2. **Psychosis and the Shattered Mirror**

Psychosis is perhaps the most feared and misunderstood of all mental states. It is often painted as a total break from reality. But when we pause to ask why someone's reality had to break in the first place, we begin to see more than chaos; we see meaning-making. It is important to note here that the symbols that emerge in psychosis—angels, demons, conspiracies, divine missions—are not random. For many survivors of trauma, especially those who were gaslit or emotionally abandoned, these symbolic narratives offer structure. They become the scaffolding for a shattered self, a bridge to coherence when language and logic fall short.

From this vantage point, psychosis may be the psyche's final attempt to reorganise meaning after unbearable rupture. It is not always something to be extinguished; sometimes, it is something to be understood.

The key takeaway here is that a trauma-informed lens doesn't reject diagnosis; it reframes it. It recognises that while clinical terms can guide treatment, they must not eclipse the person's lived truth. When we honour the story beneath the symptom, we move from pathology to possibility.

Ultimately, reframing mental disorders as trauma responses is not about romanticising suffering but about restoring dignity. It is about meeting people where they are, without fear or judgement, and saying: 'I see the logic in your experience. I trust your body's wisdom. Let's build safety here.' And when we do that, healing becomes less about fixing and more about remembering who we are, what we have endured, and what we are still capable of becoming.

Therapeutic Models for Belief Work

When clients bring supernatural experiences, spiritual encounters, or deeply rooted belief systems into therapy, it can challenge traditional therapeutic frameworks. Yet, these beliefs often carry deep personal meaning, especially for those who have lived through trauma, cultural dislocation, or identity fragmentation. As mentioned earlier, instead of dismissing or pathologising such material, many contemporary models invite us to meet it with openness, curiosity, and symbolic understanding. From this starting point, we can begin to consider how best to hold such experiences in a structured yet compassionate way.

It is also essential to recognise that there is no singular or 'correct' approach to working with belief-based or fantastical content. But over time, certain frameworks have emerged that offer structure while still respecting the depth and complexity of the inner world. These approaches aim not to debate the reality of the client's experience, but to engage with the meaning it holds for them.

The following are some of the approaches that have shown promise in navigating such content with both sensitivity and structure.

1. **Symbolic Translation**

   This approach honours the emotional and psychological truths embedded within symbolic or supernatural imagery. For instance, a demonic figure might be understood as a manifestation of internalised rage or long-buried shame. An ancestral voice could carry the weight of unspoken generational grief, or wisdom that had no other way to be heard. Therefore, instead of labelling them as hallucinations or fabrications, symbolic translation views these experiences as metaphors for wounds that were never given words.

2. **Narrative Therapy**

   Stories are how we make sense of experience. Narrative therapy treats the belief as a narrative, not to be dissected for flaws but explored for patterns, themes, and authorship. Clients are encouraged to consider: 'Who wrote this story?', 'What role am I playing?', and 'What if I could rewrite it?' This process helps individuals retain the emotional and symbolic power of their beliefs, while gaining greater agency over the story's direction.

3. **Parts Work and Internal Family Systems (IFS)**

   IFS shifts the perspective from viewing inner voices or supernatural entities as symptoms to recognising them as distinct parts of the self, each with a specific role and origin. What appears as an external spirit may be a young protector who stepped in during trauma. This model encourages respectful engagement with these parts, fostering internal dialogue, compassion, and ultimately, integration.

4. **Somatic and Polyvagal Approaches**

   Belief-based experiences are rarely just 'in the mind.' Many clients report intense physical sensations: sleep paralysis, dissociation, chronic tension, or visceral fear. Somatic therapies help clients ground themselves, attune to bodily cues, and build a felt sense of safety. Polyvagal-informed work adds nuance by helping clients understand how their nervous systems may be swinging between states of threat, shutdown, and connection and how that physiology can colour the content of belief or perception.

In all of these approaches, the therapist is not tasked with determining what is real, but rather with supporting the client in understanding why something feels real, what it might be communicating, and how to hold it in a way that brings more wholeness rather than fragmentation. Ultimately, belief work in therapy is less about resolving fantasy versus fact, and more about restoring coherence in a psyche that may have used stories, symbols, or visions to survive and now seeks to heal.

Tailoring Techniques to Personal Narratives

As was covered earlier, beliefs do not emerge in a vacuum. They are deeply shaped by personal history, cultural context, and psychological need. What one person interprets as a divine calling, another might experience as a burden, a curse, or a test. This subjectivity lies at the heart of therapeutic work with belief systems, making cultural humility and individualised attunement not just helpful, but essential.

In therapeutic practice, we often see that belief-based material cannot be approached with a one-size-fits-all methodology. Even when two clients express similar experiences—say, hearing a voice or sensing a presence—the meaning and emotional charge of those experiences can be radically different. One may feel protected or chosen; the other, haunted or condemned. These internal narratives are filtered through layers of upbringing, trauma, social conditioning, and neurological wiring.

This is why tailoring techniques to personal narratives becomes such a vital part of the healing process. It requires clinicians to go beyond diagnostic categories and into the subtle textures of a client's lived world. From a growing body of case studies and interviews, one insight stands out repeatedly: the same intervention can produce opposite effects in different clients. A ritual-based grounding exercise may bring profound peace to someone raised in a spiritual household, while the same technique may feel alien or even triggering to a client with a history of religious trauma. For some, language rooted in metaphor, archetype, or mythology can unlock powerful insights. For others, safety is built through scientific language, nervous system education, or even humour. This doesn't mean therapists need to be fluent in every tradition or belief system; it means they must remain flexible, curious, and humble. They must be willing to translate therapeutic concepts into the emotional and cognitive language their clients understand.

Above all, the goal is not to correct or invalidate a client's belief system, but to join them inside it—to understand its structure, its emotional logic, and the role it plays in their psychic survival. Within that framework, therapeutic work becomes less about dismantling and more about deep listening, slow integration, and the gentle movement towards coherence. Whether belief manifests as a symptom, a coping strategy, or a source of meaning, it deserves to be met with respect and thoughtful inquiry.

In this light, healing is not the abandonment of belief, but the transformation of the relationship to it. The therapist becomes not a judge of truth, but a witness to the deeper truths the belief may be pointing towards.

Ethical Frameworks for Belief-Oriented Therapy

Working with clients' belief systems—especially those involving supernatural, spiritual, or non-consensus realities—

requires more than clinical skill; it demands a foundation of deep ethical clarity. These beliefs often arise from complex intersections of culture, trauma, meaning-making, and survival. Mishandling them, even with good intentions, can retraumatise rather than heal.

Therapists are not required to share a client's worldview, but they are ethically obligated to engage with it respectfully. This begins with acknowledging that belief is not just content but also the structure. It organises how a person relates to their suffering, identity, agency, and even their future. Whether a client believes they are cursed, guided by ancestral spirits, or receiving messages from a higher realm, the belief itself may be less important than what it does for their nervous system and sense of coherence. Moreover, ethical attunement doesn't mean staying neutral. It means staying relational. It means meeting the client not as a fixed identity, but as a meaning-making being in motion. In this way, therapy becomes a shared process of healing.

There are several core ethical principles that help navigate this delicate terrain, as shown below:

1. **Cultural Competence Versus Cultural Appropriation**

   Therapists must recognise the fine line between appreciating a client's worldview and co-opting elements they don't fully understand. For instance, referencing indigenous rituals, chakras, or ancestral trauma without context or permission can cause harm, even if well-meaning. Cultural humility means not only being informed but being willing to step back, acknowledge limitations, and centre the client's expertise in their own traditions. Remember, curiosity is welcome, but entitlement is not.

2. **Non-Coercion**

   Therapeutic safety relies on honouring the client's agency. Clients must never feel pressured to reframe or rationalise their beliefs to align with the therapist's worldview. A client who speaks of possession, karma, or divine punishment should not be subtly coaxed into renaming their experience as psychosis, delusion, or dysregulation, unless that language resonates for them. The aim is not to impose a particular narrative, but to support the client in finding the language that makes them feel safest and most understood.

3. **Consent and Transparency**

   When therapists introduce new frames—such as symbolic interpretations or parts-based work—these should always be offered as possibilities, not prescriptions. Framing something as a metaphor may be helpful for one client but feel invalidating for another. Always ask: 'Would it feel okay if we explored this as one way of looking at it?' This leaves space for collaboration, consent, and revision.

4. **Self-Work**

   Perhaps most crucially, therapists must be in an active relationship with their own inner material. A practitioner's unresolved spiritual wounds, scepticism, awe, or discomfort can unconsciously leak into the room, shaping tone, posture, and even what gets named. Additionally, projection—whether idealisation or dismissal—can fracture trust. Ethical belief-oriented therapy requires that the therapist be aware of the filters they bring, continually asking, 'Whose meaning am I prioritising right now?'

In conclusion, when approached with care, belief-oriented therapy offers more than just symptom management. It becomes a space where personal narratives can be understood, redefined, and healed. Clients are not asked to discard what once gave them structure, nor are they trapped inside it. Instead, they are invited to re-inhabit their life story with greater choice, clarity, and dignity.

Enhancing Therapeutic Outcomes

When therapists honour a client's belief system—including those that might appear irrational, mystical, or outside the bounds of conventional understanding—they create a space where deeper healing can unfold. In such an environment, clients are not asked to fragment themselves into acceptable and unacceptable parts but are instead invited to bring their full inner world into the therapeutic space. This inclusivity fosters a profound sense of safety, which in itself becomes therapeutic.

Clients who feel seen and not pathologised often report marked shifts in their emotional and relational landscape. In sessions that allow for belief-oriented exploration—whether the content involves ancestral memories, synchronicities, spiritual visitations, or culturally embedded metaphors of illness—clients frequently experience:

- A reduction in shame and isolation, as the parts of their story that once felt too strange or too much are finally allowed to be spoken aloud.
- Increased self-compassion, as they begin to recognise that their beliefs may have developed as adaptive, meaning-making tools in the face of suffering.

- Greater access to embodied awareness, as disowned or feared experiences become integrated rather than avoided.
- The ability to speak about trauma without bypass or dissociation, since the therapeutic container no longer invalidates the language or framework they use to describe their pain.

All in all, when belief is treated as a portal rather than a problem, the therapy room transforms. The work no longer hinges on whether a belief is factually correct or clinically appropriate but instead focuses on what the belief holds, protects, or reveals. What symbolic truth might be embedded in the idea of being cursed? What internal exile is mirrored in a dream visitation? What cultural wisdom lies beneath a client's fear of breaking a taboo?

In this way, belief work is not a detour from therapy. It is often the doorway into the core story, the place where language, memory, emotion, and metaphor converge. Beliefs, no matter how unconventional, often point towards unspeakable pain or unacknowledged needs. When therapists can meet those beliefs with curiosity and attunement rather than correction or avoidance, new dimensions of healing open up.

Crucially, this approach doesn't ask clients to choose between believing themselves and healing themselves. It reframes healing as an act of deeper belief, not necessarily in the literal content but in the self who lived it, survived it, and is now ready to be witnessed. Through this lens, belief-oriented therapy becomes a reclamation of meaning, embodiment, and personal truth. This reclamation paves the way for integration of mind and body, logic and intuition, story and sensation.

On the whole, in a world that too often splits the psychological from the spiritual, the rational from the intuitive, this form of therapy says: You can be whole here.

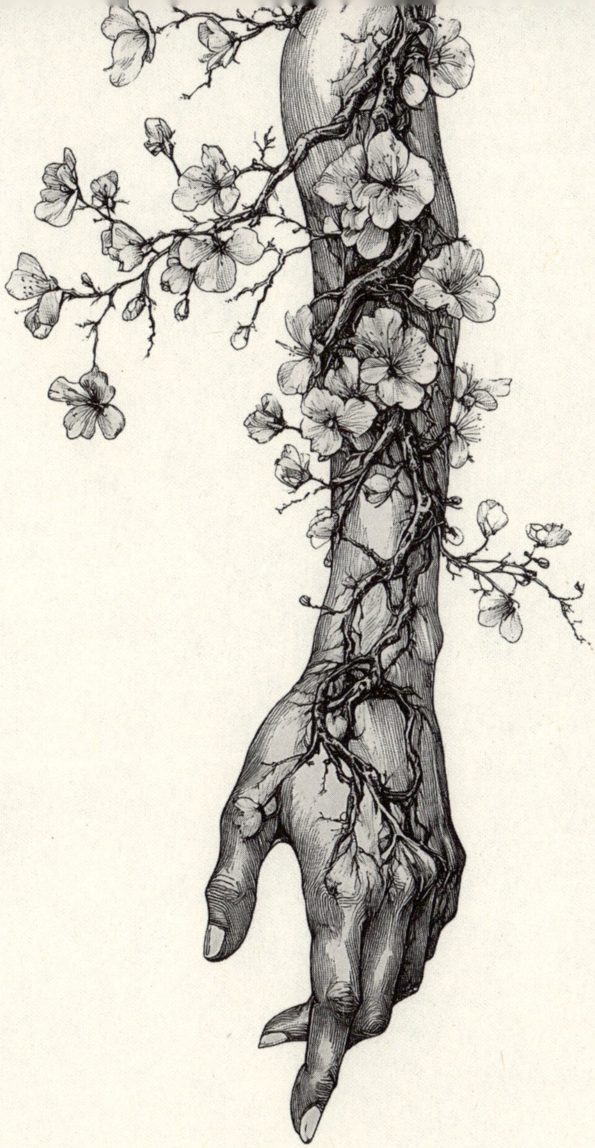

Part II
Integration and Identity

Chapter 6

Reclaiming the Child Within

'The child within us doesn't need fixing. They need to be believed, seen, and loved in the ways they never were.'

Healing the various parts of the self involves addressing the different emotional, psychological, and spiritual aspects that make up one's identity. These include the inner child, which represents past traumas or unmet needs; the feminine self, which embodies qualities like intuition, receptivity, and emotional depth; and the spiritual self, which is tied to a sense of purpose and connection. By understanding and nurturing these distinct aspects, individuals can move towards holistic well-being. For instance, healing the inner child helps release emotional pain from the past, while embracing the spiritual self can cultivate inner peace and meaning.

Readers can benefit from this understanding by learning to recognise the fragmented aspects of themselves and attending to each part's unique needs. This integrative approach can improve emotional regulation, deepen self-awareness, and enhance both mental and physical health. As these aspects are brought into harmony, individuals often experience personal growth, emotional balance, and a greater sense of fulfilment.

In this chapter, we will focus on how we can nurture and heal the inner child. Reconnecting with this vulnerable yet vital part of ourselves can lead to profound emotional release, increased self-compassion, and a more grounded sense of identity. Healing the inner child is often the first step in a larger journey of integration. In the chapters that follow, we will expand this work by exploring how to acknowledge, embrace, and harmonise the various other parts of the self, each carrying its own needs, emotions, and patterns. This process of inner integration helps us move towards wholeness, emotional resilience, and authentic self-expression.

The Child Within

The concept of an inner child features frequently across psychological schools of thought, although different disciplines tend to use different labels when referring to similar ideas. The concept originated with Jung, whose archetypes saw the inner child as a vital part of the developing personality that engages with the world while preserving a connection to imagination, curiosity, and wonder. Caroline Myss expanded on this idea by defining the inner child as the part of a person that longs for innocence, regardless of their age. She further developed this idea into sub-archetypes. For instance, the wounded child refers to those who experienced abuse or neglect in childhood. This archetype frequently appears in therapy, where clients often revisit childhood trauma as the root of their current struggles. Such individuals may wrestle with self-pity or low self-esteem and may direct blame towards their parents or loved ones for their present suffering. They may also seek out parental figures or rescuers in times of distress, rather than relying on their own inner strength or capacity to shape their reality.

Another sub-archetype, the abandoned or orphaned child, reflects individuals who experienced deep loneliness, rejection, or abandonment during their formative years. Often highly independent due to having had to fend for themselves early in life, these individuals may nevertheless carry a longing for acceptance and love. They may also struggle with embracing adult responsibilities, including forming stable, mature relationships.

The eternal child represents those who resist growing up, either by refusing to behave in ways deemed appropriate for adults or by avoiding decision-making and accountability. These individuals often have difficulty finding stability in adulthood and may prove unreliable, both to themselves and others.

The magical or innocent child sub-archetype is characterised by a persistent belief in goodness and wonder, even in the face of hardship. While these individuals tend to be optimistic, trauma can cause them to become disillusioned or cynical, potentially leading to depressive symptoms or a tendency to retreat into fantasy, under the belief that action is either unnecessary or futile.

In earlier psychoanalytic theory, Freud introduced the concept of regression, a coping mechanism in which individuals under stress revert to an earlier developmental stage. This regression may manifest in childlike behaviours, speech, or mannerisms, as the inner child rises to the surface. Jung, in contrast, viewed the inner child as the child hero, the bearer of future potential who fights life's battles and returns transformed. When a person regresses under stress, it can be seen as a summoning of this child hero, which is an inner figure called forth to protect, defend, or metaphorically slay the monster.

These archetypes frequently appear in therapeutic settings, especially as clients revisit their childhoods to make sense of the experiences that shaped them. While Freud and Jung laid the foundation for the idea of the inner child, Myss's sub-archetypes offer a more structured way to connect childhood experiences with present-day emotional and behavioural patterns. In therapeutic work, recognising which inner child is acting out can provide deep insight into the client's healing journey.

Techniques for Healing the Inner Child

The following psychological techniques help in reintegrating and healing the inner child. They also promote foundational healing by creating a sense of safety and helping one address and resolve wounds from the past.

1. **Inner Child Work**

   Inner child work involves a set of therapeutic techniques that help individuals connect with, nurture, and care for their inner child. This practice acknowledges unresolved emotional wounds from childhood and provides a way to process and heal them. Common practices include:

   - **Guided Visualisation:** A technique in which you imagine meeting, comforting, and hugging your inner child.
   - **Dialogue with the Inner Child:** Communicate directly with your inner child by asking questions or describing situations and observing what thoughts or feelings emerge.
   - **Reparenting:** Instead of ignoring or suppressing your inner child, you take on the role of the

caregiver, giving them what they once needed but didn't receive.

2. **Play Therapy and Creative Expression**

   Play therapy and creative expression significantly support the healing of the inner child. These techniques offer healthy outlets for emotions, help individuals process core wounds, and reconnect with joy. Building on this foundation, the following creative therapies offer specific and effective ways to engage with and heal the inner child through expressive, embodied experiences:

   - **Art Therapy:** It involves painting, drawing, or engaging with any other creative medium to express and explore feelings.
   - **Music Therapy:** This therapy uses music—whether through listening, singing, or playing instruments—to evoke emotions and enable emotional release.
   - **Dance and Movement Therapy:** It involves using the body through movement or dance to connect with emotions and release held or suppressed energy.

3. **Journaling**

   Journaling is a therapeutic tool that helps individuals revisit their inner child's suppressed thoughts, memories, and emotional experiences, both joyful and painful. Writing provides a space for expression, reflection, and healing, helping to normalise and process emotional wounds.

To deepen this practice, here are a few journaling prompts designed to help you connect more intimately with your inner child and uncover meaningful insights:

- Recall a happy moment from your childhood. What emotions come up? How would you describe yourself during that time?
- Write a letter to your inner child. Tell them how much they are loved and valued.
- Reflect on a threat or fear you experienced as a child. How did it impact you then? How does it affect you now?

4. **Self-Compassion and Self-Care**

   Practising self-compassion and forgiveness is essential for nurturing the inner child. This means being patient, kind, and gentle with yourself, especially when difficult emotions arise.

Guided Meditation: Reparenting Your Inner Child

This guided meditation is more than a moment of reflection; it is a powerful step towards emotional integration and self-compassion. By reparenting your inner child, you begin to shift the impact of past wounds, replacing old narratives with healing ones. It allows you to build a sense of inner security and wholeness, which strengthens your ability to navigate present-day challenges with greater clarity, resilience, and self-trust.

The following steps are designed to help you move through this guided meditation with clarity and intention.

1. **Preparation**

   Set aside 20-30 minutes in a calm, quiet environment. Sit or lie down in a comfortable position, take a deep breath, and follow the instructions with your eyes closed.

2. **Comfortable Position**

   Begin by settling into a comfortable position. Allow your muscles to relax. Let go of the tension in your shoulders, neck, arms, stomach, back, and legs. Breathe deeply and feel your body begin to soften. Close your eyes and exhale slowly a few times.

3. **Visualise Your Inner Child**

   Take a few more deep breaths. Bring to mind a place where you feel completely safe and at peace. This could be a real place or an imagined one; basically, somewhere you enjoy being. Now, in this safe space, imagine a younger version of yourself appearing. What do they look like? How do they express themselves? What is their mood? Be open and curious as you observe and approach your inner child.

4. **Provide Reassurance**

   Picture your inner child sitting near you. Imagine yourself kneeling beside them or sitting down at their level. You may choose to embrace them lovingly. Feel the warmth of this embrace and the comfort it brings to both of you. Speak to your inner child with gentleness and care. Say things like:

   - 'I love you and I will protect you.'
   - 'You are safe with me.'
   - 'I will always be here to care for you.'

5. **Healing Light**

   Now imagine a warm, radiant light surrounding both you and your inner child. This light is healing, and it soothes, restores, and dissolves distress. Visualise it reaching every part of you, including every cell, every thought, and every emotion. Let the light envelop and unify your spirit and your inner child's spirit, bringing a deep sense of wholeness.

6. **Empowerment Affirmation**

   Now, speak empowering affirmations to yourself and your inner child. Let these words sink in deeply and strengthen your sense of self:

   - 'I care for and cherish my inner child.'
   - 'My inner child is well cared for and deeply loved.'
   - 'I am one with my inner child.'
   - 'All emotional wounds are being healed and integrated.'
   - 'I accept and respect every part of who I am.'

   Repeat these affirmations as many times as you feel necessary. With each repetition, allow yourself to feel more whole, accepted, and loved.

7. **Future Visualisation**

   Now begin to visualise your future. See yourself moving forward in life, overcoming challenges, and living in alignment with your full potential. Picture yourself achieving your goals and dreams. Notice how empowered and fulfilled you feel as you do so.

8. **Closing**

   Take a few final deep breaths. Let the feelings of peace and completeness settle in. Slowly bring your awareness back to the present moment. Gently wiggle your fingers and toes. Take one or two more deep breaths, and when you're ready, open your eyes. You return feeling refreshed, centred, and empowered to steer the course of your life.

Case Study: The Inner Child as Self-Protection

Riya presented with marked regression, episodic depressive spells, and persistent fatigue. These episodes were accompanied by violent and hysterical outbursts. She had a history of suicidal ideation and had previously attempted to take their own life. Interestingly, during these episodes, she also showed a sudden inclination towards creative expression, such as watching excessive television or engaging in painting. While engaged in these activities, she became entirely absorbed, remained non-verbal, and refrained from any form of interaction.

The regression was evident in behaviour, mannerisms, speech patterns, and vocal tone—all of which mirrored those of a child under the age of ten. While Riya was fully aware of these behaviours, she expressed an inability to control or alter them. In therapeutic work, the general approach typically involves nurturing the inner child as part of the adult's healing process. However, in Riya's case, therapy involved working directly with the inner child who appeared on the surface, while the adult self remained hidden behind this protective construct.

Riya's episodes typically lasted two to three days, but the current episode had extended for over fifteen days with no signs of resolution. Atypical symptoms in this episode included erratic eating habits, fluctuating between a complete lack of appetite and episodes of binge eating.

The case history revealed regression to an age range of ten or younger, which is an important observation, as there were strong indicators of abuse, particularly sexual abuse, around this time. It was also significant that she spoke about this abuse only during episodes and refused to acknowledge or address it outside of them.

In recent years, Riya experienced additional trauma, including a suicide attempt by pill overdose. Not long after, she became pregnant and underwent an abortion at approximately three months of gestation. Curiously, she did not appear to be emotionally affected by this event and spoke of it without distress—the only trauma they were willing to discuss openly outside of an episode. It was also noted that whereas Riya had previously expressed a desire to have children, this had since changed, and they no longer felt inclined to do so.

During childhood, Riya recalled hearing voices that encouraged self-harm. These voices reportedly instructed them to go to the terrace and jump. Around the age of five, she also reported seeing faces on a curtain—an experience that triggered a pronounced freeze response. Soon after this incident, a loved one passed away, which was a loss she believed was caused by the same voices.

The fight-flight-freeze system (FFFS) provided a framework to understand such responses to trauma. It emphasised how these coping mechanisms were shaped early in life, when higher-order cognition was still underdeveloped. As such, these early responses often became embedded in one's neurological and cognitive makeup. In Riya's case, the freeze response triggered in childhood seemed to have persisted into adulthood and resurfaced in episodes involving trauma. This suggested a deeply ingrained maladaptive pattern marked by an inability to speak out or act against perceived injustice.

Riya also reported significant distress related to family dynamics. There were ongoing issues with members of their in-laws' household. Managing the home had imposed a drastic change in their sleep cycle and lifestyle, adding further stress. Moreover, the in-laws' residence was situated next to a cemetery, and the intense heat in the area often caused Riya to faint, requiring energy supplements to complete routine chores. These cumulative stressors were noted as significant contributors to her emotional and physical strain.

In discussing their family of origin, Riya described profound disappointment upon discovering that their father drank excessively and became verbally and physically abusive while intoxicated. A history of domestic violence was recorded, with the father often directing his anger towards Riya's mother. She expressed a deep sense of guilt for being unable to protect their mother from the abuse. There appeared to be a thematic link between this helplessness in childhood and her current struggle to assert themselves in the face of mistreatment, particularly from authoritative male figures towards loved female figures.

During episodes, her anger and resentment towards family members, especially her parents, intensified sharply. She became physically aggressive when her parents attempted to communicate or make physical contact. In a recent episode prior to the current one, this aggression escalated to such a degree that Riya had to be locked in a room by family members to prevent further harm.

In earlier sessions, Riya hinted at abuse from a teacher but refused to speak more about it. In later sessions, she shared that they harboured feelings of hatred towards God for allowing injustice to occur. Once again, the recurring pattern of being unable to speak up against injustice and abuse, especially when perpetrated by a respected male figure, was noted. It was also observed that Riya exhibited a diminished sense of self-worth. Her guilt and self-hatred became apparent in the way she punished herself whenever she spoke about her trauma, both through words and non-verbal cues.

Riya's regression can be interpreted as a potential fragmentation of the psyche. Not only did she revert to a childlike state, but she also became extremely aggressive and violent. The shift in personality during these episodes was dramatic, though she remained consciously present and aware throughout.

Later sessions revealed Riya's aspirations. She expressed a long-standing desire to have a career. However, after marriage, she was pushed into a domestic role, which she described as leaving her with a sense of lost purpose. She also shared dreams of travelling and opening a café. Although she briefly worked in the family business, she found it unfulfilling and chose to leave. Currently, Riya sells handmade crafts on a website her spouse created for her.

Psychotherapy, combined with hypnotherapy, was selected as the course of treatment. Given Riya's difficulty in speaking openly about the abuse and its likely connection to their presenting issues, this approach was seen as necessary to help them begin to unpack their experiences and emotions. During these sessions, she disclosed that they had been sexually assaulted by a teacher over a span of two years. A strong link is drawn between this incident and her persistent feelings of guilt, self-hatred, and helplessness in the face of injustice. It also relates to her deep emotional responses to scenarios involving respected male figures harming beloved female figures.

At this stage, it becomes evident that Riya embodies the archetype of the wounded child—someone who has suffered abuse or neglect and holds their parents responsible for their pain. Her violent outbursts towards their parents during episodes and her difficulty relating to her spouse's parents were likely rooted in these early experiences of betrayal. The wounded child is also associated with issues of low self-esteem and self-pity, both of which are clearly present in Riya's case. Additionally, individuals in this archetype often depend on parental figures rather than take responsibility for themselves. In Riya's case, this has taken a more literal form, where they regress into a childlike state requiring care and protection from others.

Riya's therapy incorporated visualisation and guided imagery, along with roleplay and imaginative projection. In one exercise, she imagined confronting her abuser in the presence of God, compelling the abuser to confess and visualising their punishment. This process helped her release repressed emotions and begin to process their trauma. She also participated in the empty chair technique, engaging in imagined conversations with deceased loved ones. This practice gradually gave her the space to say goodbye and begin grieving these losses. Such visualisation and enactment techniques are powerful tools for meaning-making in the aftermath of trauma, allowing clients to consolidate their emotional experiences and form what is known as a 'continuing bond' with the deceased.

When discussing family further, Riya shares that her siblings constantly criticised her, and she felt like a failure, always having to prove herself to those around them. She expressed a belief that she was destined to fail at everything. Once again, there was a pronounced sense of self-hatred and guilt, this time linked to their perceived inability to follow through on goals or meet external expectations. Additionally, Riya described a range of interpersonal issues among family members, suggesting that their home environment is riddled with multiple ongoing stressors.

When reflecting on her other parent, Riya stated that she was emotionally distant—unable to express love—and professionally unsuccessful. She described feeling caged or trapped in their circumstances, accompanied by a strong urge to break free. It appeared that she also embodied traits of the abandoned or orphaned child—someone who felt isolated and unloved, and who was often forced to take on the role of their own caretaker. Riya's deep-rooted self-hatred stemmed from this early emotional neglect and the chronic feeling of being rejected or criticised. Her tendency to regress might also be connected to these formative experiences, as she was compelled to grow up too soon, both due to trauma and the necessity of emotional self-reliance.

As therapy progressed, Riya's regression began to subside, and she became more coherent in sessions. She expressed that the emotional release, particularly around the abuse, felt like a weight had been lifted. Therapeutic work continued, focusing on releasing suppressed emotions and helping her move towards resolution and integration.

Following this emotional breakthrough, Riya stated that she believed a relative had cursed her with black magic. It became increasingly evident that her locus of control remained largely external. With each psychological layer that was uncovered, there appeared to be a different entity or force representing this external control. Her concept of power also seemed distorted as she tended to associate strength with authoritative, often male, figures, while viewing herself and women in general as being controlled or subjugated. A subconscious vow seemed to have formed: Riya's belief that men are abusers and women are victims had become the lens through which they interpreted her relationships and the world at large. In most of her relationships with men, some form of abuse was present, while with women, she tended to find emotional safety and support.

While Riya does have a support system in the women around them, she lacks anyone in her life who models healthy strength or agency. As a result, the focus of her treatment was to help her recognise and begin to cultivate her own inner strength. Trauma therapy in such cases must take into account that the abusers may still be part of the client's daily life, i.e., present during the healing process and likely beyond. Therefore, the treatment plan should include strategies to build emotional resilience and develop coping mechanisms in anticipation of potential future encounters with their abusers.

Riya's healing journey was layered and complex, involving multiple sub-archetypes that manifest through severe regression. While notable improvements were observed in her symptoms, it is clear that healing will require time and patience as she gradually confronts and works through each layer of trauma.

Chapter 7

Connecting with the Feminine Self

'The feminine self is not something to become, but something we remember. It is an inner knowing we were taught to forget.'

The concept of femininity is relatively new in psychology, largely because much of the earlier literature focused on male experiences and, in doing so, masculinised the self. Later theorists such as Freud and Jung viewed the self as existing between conscious expression and the subconscious mind. Jung further described the self as an archetype that integrates all aspects of consciousness, including elements of other archetypes. However, the exclusion of female experiences—and, by extension, feminine traits—renders such integration incomplete, as it overlooks essential dimensions of human personality.

Traditional views of the self emphasised the rational mind and placed value on agency, consciousness, and logic, often at the cost of excluding women's selfhood and experiences of emotion and creativity as integral to self-expression. Modern psychology has gradually expanded to include feminist perspectives, which recognise the self as influenced by a broader range of factors, including femininity. Though femininity is culturally associated with women, it comprises a spectrum of traits that are not exclusive to any one gender. Engaging with this dimension of the personality is an important aspect of healing and of forming a more integrated, authentic sense of self.

Working with femininity allows for an understanding of the self as complex, interconnected, and fluid. This approach creates space in therapy to address deeply personal and emotionally nuanced issues such as intimacy, rejection, isolation, abuse, and sexual trauma. These experiences are often accompanied by complex emotions such as shame and guilt, and healing from them requires vulnerability, self-compassion, and emotional expression.

By integrating all aspects of the self—including the feminine—without shame, individuals are offered the opportunity to take ownership of their healing journey, acknowledge their inner power, and work towards wholeness.

Disconnection from the Feminine Self

In a world that often glorifies productivity, logic, and external validation, many individuals—regardless of gender—find themselves distanced from the softer, more intuitive dimensions of their being. The feminine self, which embodies qualities such as receptivity, emotional wisdom, inner knowing, and relational depth, is not limited to any one identity; it is a vital inner compass that helps us feel whole, nourished, and connected.

Disconnection from this feminine essence doesn't happen overnight. It is often the result of cultural conditioning, survival strategies, or past wounding that taught us to silence our feelings, override our intuition, and measure our worth by output alone. Over time, this separation can manifest in subtle but persistent ways such as emotional numbness, chronic burnout, strained relationships, and a sense of inner hollowness. Recognising the signs of this disconnection is the first step toward reclaiming a more balanced and integrated self.

Signs that one may be disconnected from their feminine self include:

1. **Intuitive Blankness:** Inability to listen to or trust inner guidance.
2. **Emotional Disconnect:** Difficulty identifying emotions or relating empathetically to others.
3. **Burnout Syndrome:** Focusing only on achievement and external success while neglecting self-care and emotional nourishment.
4. **Detached Relationships:** Lack of emotional depth and support within personal connections.

Integration of the Feminine Self

The process of realising and integrating one's feminine self involves identifying, accepting, and safeguarding this essential part of identity. This journey of reintegration requires courage, compassion, and the willingness to cherish a core aspect of who we are.

Reconnecting with the feminine self begins by making space for intuition, emotion, and receptivity—qualities that are often silenced in environments driven by constant productivity or perfectionism. It means listening inward rather than constantly seeking validation from outside. For some, this might look like honouring emotional needs without judgement. For others, it may mean slowing down enough to hear the quiet wisdom beneath the noise of daily life.

As this inner relationship deepens, the feminine self begins to feel safe enough to emerge. We start to relate to ourselves with greater softness and to others with greater empathy. This process does not require abandoning ambition or strength, but balancing them with nourishment, presence, and self-trust. True integration is not about conforming to an ideal of femininity, but about reclaiming the parts of ourselves that allow us to feel, flow, and belong within and without.

Ways to Engage with the Feminine Self

There are several ways in which individuals can connect with their feminine self and begin to embody its qualities. Engaging with creativity—through art, music, dance, or journaling—can help open channels to the inner feminine. Additionally, practices that cultivate receptivity and stillness, such as meditation, mindful movement, or spending time in nature, are also deeply supportive. Fostering nurturing relationships and exploring vulnerability in safe spaces can also allow people to soften their defences and build trust in their inner wisdom. Over time, this conscious engagement can help restore balance, wholeness, and emotional resilience.

Given below are some helpful techniques and practices to engage with the feminine side of oneself.

1. **Meditation**

   Meditative techniques can help clients access their creative, intuitive, and emotional selves, deepening their connection with the feminine self.

2. **Journaling**

   Writing about personal experiences—particularly those related to feminine qualities—can support emotional processing and insight. Journaling provides a safe outlet for expression and discovery.

Here are a few journaling prompts to support a deeper connection with your inner feminine self.

- Recall a moment when you felt deeply connected to your intuition. What did it feel like?
- Reflect on someone you have nurtured, whether a child, pet, or loved one. How did the experience affect both of you?
- Write a letter to your feminine self. Express your appreciation for her and your desire to grow into her nurturing presence.

3. **Accept Femininity**

Acknowledge and embrace inner traits commonly regarded as feminine, such as intuition, compassion, and nurturing. Recognise these not as weaknesses but as strengths that support well-being and balance.

- **Intuition:** Pay attention to internal cues and gut feelings. Trust your instincts rather than dismissing them in favour of over-rationalisation.
- **Empathy:** Empathy involves listening to emotional pain—your own and others'—and responding with compassion, not just understanding.
- **Nurturing:** Actively care for yourself and others. Engage in behaviours that promote emotional nourishment, kindness, and connection.

4. **Create and Use Expressive Arts**

   Engaging with the arts can be a powerful way to access and express the feminine self. These activities allow emotions to surface and be processed in a healthy, creative way. Use painting, music, dance, or other forms of expression to give voice to feelings and reconnect with the softer, intuitive side of yourself.

5. **Practice Self-Reflection**

   Carve out time regularly to reflect inwardly. This helps strengthen your relationship with the feminine archetype and allows you to consciously integrate its qualities into your everyday life. Such self-reflection sessions involve setting aside time each week for introspection and exploring how you can invite more feminine energy—such as intuition, softness, or emotional openness—into your thoughts and actions.

Guided Meditation: Embracing the Feminine Self

The guided visualisation given below has been designed to help individuals reconnect with, reclaim, and nurture their inner feminine self. This aspect of the self often holds the energy of intuition, creativity, receptivity, compassion, and emotional depth, which are qualities that may be suppressed or overlooked in daily life. By consciously engaging with this part of oneself, individuals can cultivate greater balance, self-acceptance, and inner harmony.

The following steps will guide you through the process.

1. **Preparation**

   Find a comfortable and safe space where you can remain undisturbed for 20 to 30 minutes. Sit or lie down in a position that feels most relaxed. When ready, gently close your eyes and relax your back, shoulders, and neck. Take a few slow, deep breaths, inhaling through your nose and holding gently for a few seconds. Then, exhale softly through your mouth. With each breath, imagine tension melting from your muscles and your mind clearing. Allow your attention to settle gently at the centre of your forehead, bringing clarity and stillness.

2. **Picture Feminine Energy**

   Continue breathing mindfully. Now imagine a soft, maternal light—a symbol of feminine energy—surrounding you. Visualise it enveloping your body, filling you with warmth and compassion. Feel this gentle light moving through each cell, embracing and healing every part of you with tender presence.

3. **Honour Feminine Qualities**

   Bring to mind the qualities often associated with the feminine: tenderness, empathy, compassion, guidance, and emotional wisdom. Visualise orbs of light within you growing stronger with each breath, representing these traits. Tune into your intuition, your capacity to nurture, and your ability to hold space for vulnerability and healing.

4. **Affirmations**

   In your mind's eye, repeat the following affirmations slowly, allowing their meaning to sink in with feeling and intention:

- 'I greet and welcome the feminine energy within me.'
- 'I am kind-hearted and trust my intuition.'
- 'I honour the divine feminine aspect of my being.'
- 'I love and care deeply for myself and others.'
- 'I am whole, complete, and in balance.'

Repeat these affirmations once in the morning and again before bed. With each repetition, allow your sense of confidence, self-love, and inner connection to grow stronger.

5. **Healing Light**

   Visualise a warm, radiant light surrounding and filling you completely. Imagine this healing light as a nurturing energy that touches every part of you, including your cells, thoughts, emotions, and spirit. Feel it bringing harmony and reintegration to all aspects of your being.

6. **Future Visualisation**

   See yourself moving through life with grace and assurance. Visualise yourself confidently facing challenges, embracing opportunities, and fulfilling your goals. Feel yourself stepping fully into your purpose and potential, empowered by your connection to your feminine self.

Case Study: Control and the Feminine Self

Tara presented with ongoing struggles around weight loss. In addition to physical concerns such as gastric issues, migraines, and breathing difficulties, she reported emotional and psychological distress, including anxiety, suicidal thoughts, and bulimic behaviours.

Tara described herself as someone who suppressed emotions, particularly sorrow, and was often overwhelmed by anxiety and a sense of emotional isolation. She described her spouse as short-tempered and prone to depression and anxiety. This created a dynamic in which Tara felt she had to constantly remain cautious and could not freely express herself.

The feminine quality of emotional self-expression has historically been devalued. At one point, it was even pathologised; women who showed strong emotions were often diagnosed with hysteria and treated accordingly. While this perspective was no longer medically accepted, the social stigma around emotional openness—especially emotions deemed feminine—still persisted. In Tara's case, this stigma resulted in a strong internal pressure to repress her feelings out of fear and hypervigilance.

As therapy progressed, Tara began to open up about her difficulty with asserting herself. She also shared that she lacked close social connections and did not have a support system with whom she could confide. In many ways, she felt emotionally and socially restricted, unable to speak up for herself and without a safe outlet for sharing what she was experiencing.

From a mind-body perspective, unprocessed emotional pain was sometimes believed to manifest as physical issues, including excess weight. When traditional weight-loss efforts failed, it became important to explore the emotional and psychological roots of the issue. Tara described a strained relationship with food, stating that she derived no pleasure from eating and often purged after meals. Purging served as a form of catharsis—a physical release in lieu of an emotional one.

This emotional restriction and self-denial acted as a protective insulation, i.e., a way of avoiding responsibility for one's future. Maladaptive behaviours like bingeing and purging served as coping strategies that delayed the confrontation of deeper emotional wounds. Tara expressed a belief that she would only be able to address those issues after she lost weight. Therapy, therefore, focused on helping her access and express the emotions she had long suppressed. This emotional purging was framed as essential for healing and a key to releasing her unhealthy coping mechanisms.

A significant therapeutic goal for Tara was learning to stand up for herself. Naming this aloud appeared to catalyse change. Within the first few sessions, she reported beginning to enjoy food again, especially healthier options like salads and soups, which she had previously struggled to keep down. She also noted feeling more confident in managing emotional conflicts at home and stated that she had started expressing herself more openly. This shift suggested that as Tara connected more deeply with her feminine self and through emotional expression and reclaiming her voice, she began to experience both emotional and physical healing.

However, at this stage of therapy, Tara stated that she believed certain members of her extended family had cursed her using black magic. Given her presenting issues, an external locus of control was to be expected. However, what stood out was that conversations around being cursed or strongly controlled by an external force emerged most when the sessions began to focus on emotional release and self-expression. Upon further discussion, Tara revealed that she believed black magic was to blame for the problems in her marriage, and that it had also contributed to her health issues, childlessness, frequent arguments, and ongoing emotional turmoil at home. So, when therapy began addressing Tara's self-expression within the context of her marital difficulties, the theme of black magic and overpowering external forces surfaced more prominently.

Previously, Tara had deferred taking charge of her life until after she lost weight. Now, that goal had shifted again—this time, she stated that she first needed to deal with the effects of black magic. Once again, she was insulating herself from directly confronting her emotional pain and inner conflicts.

The process of emotional release and healing was expanded to include forgiveness, both of the self and of those Tara believed had wished harm upon her and her spouse. She was guided through visual imagery exercises where she imagined cutting cords that bound her and her spouse to those holding ill will towards them and was encouraged to begin the process of forgiving these individuals. Additionally, she was encouraged to engage in simple shared activities with her spouse, such as going shopping together.

A few sessions later, Tara reported that her home environment felt much more peaceful. She expressed feeling as though she had been released from the influence of black magic and shared that she was now forming new friendships with people she genuinely liked and trusted. It was observed that spending more quality time together helped the couple experience greater harmony and emotional openness in their relationship.

The emotional release work continued over the next few sessions, targeting smaller, yet significant, areas where Tara felt held back. A major focus was placed on her relationship with food. Eventually, she reported having lost one and a half kilograms of weight and, more significantly, expressed joy that the weight loss had occurred through developing a healthy, enjoyable relationship with food. She shared that she was now eating nourishing meals and actually looking forward to them.

Tara also noted visible improvements in her spouse's behaviour; he had begun releasing pent-up anger and appeared to be much calmer and less short-tempered. She shared that her spouse, too, was starting to work through his own emotional pain and fears, leading to a healthier, more positive dynamic between them.

At this point, a new layer was added to Tara's therapeutic journey: guiding her to shift her locus of control to an internal space of empowerment. Visualisation exercises were introduced to help her feel safe and protected, not just from black magic, but also from the emotional harm caused by those around her, particularly certain family members. The goal was to help her explore what she truly wanted for herself and her life, independent of external interference or emotional turbulence.

Tara shared that releasing so much emotional weight in prior sessions had left her with a sense of emptiness—a void where she had long stored pain and unexpressed feelings. She was encouraged to start filling this space by developing consistent habits aligned with a healthy and positive life. It was emphasised that it takes a minimum of twenty-one days to form a new habit, and that consistency would be key to sustaining her growth. In addition, she was guided through a visualisation technique known as the basement exercise, where clients are asked to imagine themselves in a basement and describe what they see. This technique allowed clients to symbolically project their subconscious thoughts, feelings, and desires into a visual scene. The basement itself was viewed as a metaphor for the subconscious mind, with what was stored in it representing hidden emotions or memories. Tara described seeing a child and expressed the belief that she would finally have a child that year. This visualisation was used as a springboard to help her process and release emotions related to her struggles with infertility, as well as any fears or hopes she had about future parenthood.

In the final sessions, Tara shared that her weight loss journey was continuing in a healthy, balanced way. She no longer felt anxious around the weighing scale and had stopped checking her weight obsessively. She was eating nourishing food and genuinely enjoying her meals, reflecting a far healthier relationship with food. Emotionally, she reported significant progress as she felt more stable, and her relationship with her spouse had grown stronger and more open. Her spouse, in turn, had also become more emotionally available and communicative.

This case was particularly compelling in how it vividly illustrated the concept of emotional baggage—a term that refers to the psychological and emotional weight one carries long after the original source of trauma or stress has passed. Emotional baggage could stem from childhood wounds, past traumas, or unresolved relational or professional conflicts. Over time, it could leave a person feeling stuck in repetitive cycles of thought and behaviour. And this was the case with Tara. For her, the path to healing and lasting lifestyle change involved actively addressing and releasing this emotional baggage, allowing for growth, self-empowerment, and forward movement.

Chapter 8

Integrating the Spiritual Self

'True integration happens when spirituality is not placed above the self but woven into it.'

In many therapeutic settings, the spiritual dimension of healing is often viewed as too abstract, too subjective, or too personal to belong in clinical conversation. And yet, time and again, clients arrive with questions that point beyond the realm of psychology: 'What is the purpose of my pain?', 'Who am I beyond my trauma?', and 'Is there more to me than this body, this mind, this story?' These are not just existential musings; they are invitations. Invitations to see healing not just as symptom relief, but as soul retrieval.

To integrate the spiritual self is not to impose belief, but to create space for what is already seeking expression. For some, this might look like reimagining their relationship with God, the universe, or the unknown. For others, it might be about reconnecting with awe, meaning, and a sense of inner sanctity long buried under shame, fear, or disconnection. When clients are given permission to name and engage with this part of themselves—however they define it—therapy becomes more than a container for survival. It becomes a space for expansion.

This chapter explores the many ways spiritual integration can support deep, embodied healing. It also looks at how the body can serve as a spiritual ally and how embracing the sacred—

however one understands it—can restore a sense of wholeness, even in the midst of uncertainty.

The Psychology of Spiritual Connection

Within each of us exists a spiritual self—a quiet, enduring presence that is less about religion and more about essence. It is the part of us that feels connected to something larger, whether that is nature, humanity, the universe, or a sense of the sacred that defies definition. This self often carries our deepest values, our longing for meaning, and our capacity for awe. It is not bound by the demands of daily life or the narratives we've been given about who we are. Instead, it is rooted in a timeless awareness, one that holds both our fragility and our vastness.

Yet for many, this spiritual self becomes distant, even invisible. Modern life rewards productivity over presence, certainty over wonder, and consumption over contemplation. Add to this the wounds of betrayal, loss, or disillusionment, especially if tied to spiritual traditions, and it is no surprise that we learn to turn away from this inner dimension. We begin to mistake busyness for purpose, validation for meaning, and survival for living. Over time, the voice of the spiritual self grows faint, not because it has left us, but because we have stopped listening.

The truth is that reconnecting with the spiritual self is not a luxury; it is essential to becoming whole. Without it, we risk living only from the mind or the body, cut off from the deeper currents that give life coherence. Integrating the spiritual self restores balance, aligning our inner world with our outer actions. It offers a compass when logic falters, a source of strength when life fractures, and a reminder that even in our most solitary moments, we are part of something greater. In reclaiming this part of ourselves, we do not turn away from reality but instead learn to meet it with depth, resilience, and grace.

The Inner Compass for Life's Uncertainty

Much research has attempted to empirically explore the relationship between the human mind and what is often called the spirit or soul. In essence, it is a search for a new archetype, the spiritual self. In modern literature, figures such as physician and endocrinologist Deepak Chopra have written extensively about the intersection of faith and medicine, framing it as a central element of modern healing and therapy. While such writings often fall outside conventional academic frameworks, it is worth noting that the therapeutic practices they recommend—such as meditation, mindfulness, and healthy lifestyle habits—are increasingly accepted in mainstream therapeutic work. Moreover, this body of literature offers compelling insights into how a person's faith can serve as a vital anchor, helping them hold on to hope in the face of trauma.

The spiritual self, in this context, is not bound by dogma or confined to religious identity. Rather, it represents the aspect of the human psyche that seeks connection, meaning, and coherence in the face of life's complexity. It can be expressed through prayer or ritual, but also through art, music, nature, acts of service, and quiet moments of contemplation. What unites these expressions is not the form they take, but the inner orientation they cultivate, i.e., a felt sense of belonging to something greater than oneself. This orientation has been shown to foster resilience, offering a perspective that can transcend immediate suffering and provide a sense of continuity, even in moments of deep uncertainty.

Yet, in our increasingly secular, fast-paced world, the spiritual self is often neglected or dismissed as irrelevant.

The languages of efficiency and productivity tend to crowd out the slower, subtler forms of knowing that the spiritual self speaks. For some, disconnection may also stem from disillusionment, perhaps with religious institutions, spiritual leaders, or personal experiences that left wounds instead of solace. In these cases, the spiritual self may retreat further, its voice muted by protective silence. The paradox is that the very times we feel most cut off from this inner dimension are often the times we most need it, for it holds the capacity to transform isolation into belonging, chaos into meaning, and pain into purpose.

Therapeutic integration of the spiritual self does not mean prescribing a particular belief system; it means creating space for clients to explore and define this part of themselves in their own language. It invites curiosity about where they find a sense of awe, what gives them meaning, and how they connect to something beyond the self. This process can become a powerful catalyst for healing, as it taps into resources that extend beyond rational problem-solving. These are resources that can sustain, guide, and inspire transformation long after the therapy room is left behind.

Pathways to the Spiritual Self

There are many pathways to reconnect with the spiritual self, each offering an opportunity to explore meaning, belonging, and inner peace. While the form may differ from person to person, ranging from traditional prayer to silent walks in nature, the goal remains the same, which is to awaken a sense of connection to something greater than oneself. By engaging in practices that cultivate stillness, wonder, and gratitude, we allow the spiritual dimension of our being to emerge from beneath the noise of everyday life. This conscious integration can foster resilience, deepen self-understanding, and restore a sense of purpose.

Given below are some helpful techniques and practices to engage with your spiritual self.

1. **Meditation and Contemplative Prayer**

   Quiet, intentional stillness allows the mind to settle and the deeper self to surface. Whether through silent meditation, breath awareness, or contemplative prayer, these practices can create a direct sense of connection to the spiritual dimension.

2. **Journaling for Spiritual Insight**

   Writing can be a profound tool for exploring beliefs, spiritual experiences, and questions of meaning. Journaling provides a safe space to engage with both doubt and faith, allowing you to clarify your spiritual identity.

   Here are a few prompts to explore your spiritual self:

   - Recall a time you felt part of something larger than yourself. What sensations or emotions did you experience?
   - Reflect on a moment when life felt particularly meaningful or guided. What did you take from that experience?
   - Write a letter to your spiritual self, expressing gratitude and curiosity about the journey ahead.

3. **Engage in Awe-Inspiring Experiences**

   The spiritual self often awakens in the presence of beauty, wonder, and mystery. Seek out experiences—such as witnessing a sunrise, visiting a sacred site, or immersing yourself in art or music—that evoke a sense of awe. These moments bypass rational thought and connect directly to the soul.

4. **Practice Gratitude and Mindful Presence**

   Spiritual awareness grows when we shift our focus from what is lacking to what is present. Regularly noting what you are grateful for and truly savouring the present moment can help cultivate a sense of abundance and connection to life as it is.

5. **Explore Symbolism, Ritual, and Sacred Space**

   Symbolic acts—such as lighting a candle, creating a personal altar, or performing a meaningful ritual—can anchor spiritual intention in physical form. Similarly, carving out a quiet, beautiful space for reflection can signal to the mind and body that you are entering sacred territory.

Guided Meditation: Connecting with the Spiritual Self

The guided visualisation below is designed to help individuals reconnect with and integrate their spiritual self, the part of our being that senses meaning, unity, and connection beyond the physical world. This aspect often holds the energy of presence, awe, compassion, inner peace, and trust in life's unfolding. Yet, in the busyness and demands of daily life, it can become overlooked or overshadowed. By consciously engaging with this part of ourselves, we open the door to greater clarity, purpose, and inner wholeness.

The following steps will guide you through the process.

1. **Preparation**

   Find a quiet, comfortable space where you can be free from interruptions for 20 to 30 minutes. Sit or lie down in a position that supports relaxation. Close your eyes gently, allowing your facial muscles to soften. Begin with slow, deep breaths. Inhale through your nose, hold softly for a moment, and exhale through your mouth. With each breath, imagine releasing tension, worries, and mental clutter. Allow your awareness to drop into your heart space, as if you are arriving home to yourself.

2. **Picture Spiritual Energy**

   Continue to breathe deeply and evenly. Now imagine a radiant, luminous light above you—a pure and expansive energy that represents your spiritual self. See it descending gently, enveloping you in a sphere of peace, warmth, and unconditional acceptance. Feel this light flowing into your body, bringing stillness to your mind and a sense of sacredness to your whole being.

3. **Honour Spiritual Qualities**

   Bring to mind the qualities often associated with the spiritual self: presence, compassion, trust, forgiveness, and a deep sense of connection to all life. Visualise these qualities as glowing streams of light within you, growing brighter with every breath. Sense your place in the greater tapestry of existence and feel your heart expanding with gratitude for simply being alive.

4. **Affirmations**

   In your mind's eye, repeat the following affirmations slowly, letting their truth resonate within you:

   - 'I am connected to the source of life and wisdom.'
   - 'I trust the unfolding of my journey.'
   - 'I honour the sacred within me and in all living beings.'
   - 'I am guided, supported, and at peace.'
   - 'I am whole, complete, and in harmony with the universe.'

   Repeat these affirmations in the morning and before sleep, allowing them to deepen your connection to your spiritual self over time.

5. **Healing Light**

   Visualise the luminous light around you becoming even brighter and warmer, filling every cell of your body with vitality and love. See it dissolving all fear, doubt, and disconnection. Imagine this light radiating from your heart outward, touching the world around you with kindness and compassion.

6. **Future Visualisation**

   Picture yourself moving through life with a calm, grounded presence, meeting challenges with faith and responding to others with compassion. See yourself walking with a clear sense of purpose, confident in your inner guidance, and deeply connected to the spiritual essence that has always been within you.

Case Study: Faith and Healing the Mind

Faith, spirituality, religion, and the belief in a higher power often play a significant role in healing. On one hand, this can reflect an external locus of control—the belief that an outside force governs life's events. On the other, faith can be a powerful protective factor for many individuals, providing them with strength and hope in times of suffering.

The belief that a divine or benevolent force is guiding events for the greater good can be deeply comforting. It gives individuals a framework through which they can make sense of pain, loss, and change. However, this same belief can also become a source of internal conflict when individuals are faced with intense suffering or trauma. In such moments, they may struggle to reconcile how a loving higher power could allow such pain to occur and persist.

One such case involved a client diagnosed with conversion disorder who was grappling with a loss of faith. Naina, who had once been deeply devout, had developed a sudden and intense aversion to religion. This shift appeared inexplicable at first, until sessions gradually uncovered a long history of sexual abuse that Naina had endured at her madrasa over several years. This abuse was not isolated as it extended to other students as well, and what compounded her trauma was being used as a shield to protect the abuser whenever questions arose.

Childhood trauma had a profound effect on emotional and psychological development, shaping one's ability to love and trust, worldview, and perception of justice and authority. Naina embodied the wounded child archetype, blaming God for the injustice she had endured. In Naina's internal narrative, God became akin to a neglectful parent who was meant to protect her but had failed.

Naina's inner conflict stemmed from the inability to reconcile the idea of a loving, just higher power with the brutal reality of her abuse. The trauma of childhood assault coloured her perception of all subsequent pain. For instance, she interpreted the death of a loved one as God deliberately taking someone away. Misfortunes in daily life were attributed to being cursed or targeted by black magic.

A combination of psychodynamic and gestalt approaches was used to help Naina access her childhood trauma and begin externalising the pain she had long internalised. Since her abuser was never brought to justice, this unhealed wound became a permanent ache. Instead of confronting it, Naina channelled her pain into blaming God or external supernatural forces. This allowed her to remain in the familiar role of the victim. As long as the responsibility for her suffering rested with an outside entity, Naina could avoid the heavy burden of taking ownership of her healing journey. Thus, her struggle was not only about reconciling cognitive dissonance between faith and trauma but also about how her external locus of control functioned as a defence mechanism, shielding her from engaging with the process of change.

In contrast to this, another client, Sneha, embarked on a healing journey that took on a distinctly spiritual dimension. After experiencing marital problems and being separated from her newborn child, Sneha spiralled into a period of emotional and psychological distress. Her case history revealed a deep-rooted fear of abandonment, suggesting that Sneha embodied the orphaned child archetype, i.e., struggling with feelings of rejection and burdened by guilt and fear over potentially having abandoned her own family.

As therapy progressed, Sneha began exploring philosophical and existential questions, including the nature of life and death. She shared that such conversations brought clarity in times when life felt chaotic or meaningless. Through these discussions, Sneha found comfort in spiritual perspectives and began to see endings not as final, but as the start of something new. Separation, in this light, became a temporary state rather than a permanent loss.

Sneha viewed life as a kind of drama in which humans were actors, and reality as something shaped by belief. Despite having developed a new spiritual faith, she believed that individuals created their own experiences, signifying a strong internal locus of control. This stood in stark contrast to Naina's case, where faith had represented an external authority. For Sneha, faith became a source of empowerment rather than helplessness. Her inner child began to embody the magical or innocent child archetype, showing wonder and hope even in difficult times and holding faith in a better tomorrow.

Sneha's focus in therapy soon shifted towards a spiritual path of healing. She began to accept what had happened as unchangeable and shifted her energy toward what she could influence, directing her efforts towards transforming her emotional responses to the past. Sneha practised letting go and moving forward, choosing to accept what was out of her control and invest in what was not. Her faith and spirituality formed the foundation of her therapeutic journey and became the cornerstone upon which she began to rebuild a meaningful and self-directed life.

Chapter 9

From Many Selves to One

'Inside us live countless voices, but harmony begins when they discover the same song.'

Human beings are far more intricate than a single label, role, or identity can capture. We each hold within us a constellation of parts—some familiar, some hidden, some emerging only in specific moments. Alongside the inner child, the feminine self, and the spiritual self, there may be the achiever, the rebel, the caretaker, the sceptic, the dreamer, the wounded protector, and countless others. These parts are shaped by our histories, our environments, and the stories we have told ourselves in order to survive and belong. Together, they form a rich inner landscape that is complex, multi-layered, and at times even contradictory.

While each part carries its own purpose, living with too many disconnected selves can feel like being pulled in different directions at once. One part may urge you to take bold risks, another to retreat into safety. One may cling to old wounds, while another is desperate to move forward. This internal dissonance can leave us feeling scattered, stuck, or unsure of who we really are beneath it all.

This chapter invites you into the gentle but profound work of integration, i.e., bringing these parts into dialogue, understanding their roles, and allowing them to rest within a unified sense of self. It is vital to note here that integration is not about erasing or silencing these selves, but about weaving them into a coherent whole, where each part is honoured yet no longer isolated. It is a process of creating an inner home where each self has a place, yet no single part has to carry the whole burden of living. In this way, we move from being ruled by many selves to living as one whole, authentic self.

Uniting the Self

Integrating the many parts of ourselves is not a one-time act, but an ongoing practice of attention, compassion, and balance. Just as a symphony requires each instrument to be tuned and attuned to the others, our inner life flourishes when all aspects of the self—wounded and wise, tender and strong—are heard and valued. By consciously engaging in practices that promote connection, reflection, and support, we create the conditions for these parts to work together in harmony, allowing us to live from a place of greater wholeness and authenticity.

1. **Promote Wholeness Among Different Parts of the Self**

   Begin by building a sense of communion with yourself, understanding that you are a collective of various parts, some of which may require healing. Practices such as mindfulness, meditation, and expressive arts (like art, music, and dance) can help you tune in to your internal world and cultivate a sense of convergenc and equilibrium.

   - **Mindfulness Practice**

     Take a few minutes each day to engage in mindfulness. This could be through brisk walking or simply sitting in silence. Sit comfortably and close your eyes. Pay gentle attention to your breath, your thoughts, your feelings, and bodily sensations, observing them in a detached manner. If your attention drifts, gently bring it back to your breath.

- **Meditation Practice**

  Choose a form of meditation that resonates with you—for example, transcendental meditation or loving-kindness meditation—and commit to practising it daily. Make it a part of your routine to spend time in silence, connecting with your inner self.

- **Expressive Arts**

  Creative expression is a powerful way to release emotions and thoughts. Whether it is painting, sketching, composing, singing, or moving rhythmically, such activities support emotional processing and self-understanding.

2. **Regular Self-Reflection**

   Self-reflection is a crucial part of integration and should be undertaken regularly. Embrace every aspect of yourself, including your physical, mental, emotional, and spiritual dimensions. Through reflection, you gain insight into your thoughts, behaviours, and life experiences.

   - **Journaling**

     Maintaining a journal allows you to record your thoughts, emotions, the 'whys' behind them, and significant events. Reflect on how each part of yourself weighs upon and interacts with the others. Write down your ideas, frustrations, and victories to gain clarity on your progress and inner journey.

- **Meditative Reflection**

  Sit in silence and reflect deeply. Explore the different dimensions of your being and ask yourself: 'What am I experiencing physically, emotionally, mentally, and spiritually?' and 'What does each of these aspects need in order to come into balance?'

3. **Seek Support**

   Sometimes healing requires guidance. A therapist can walk alongside you as you piece together the fragmented aspects of your self. Much of our pain stems from emotions that were never fully processed and which continue to affect the quality of our lives.

   - **Therapeutic Support**

     Look for a practitioner with a holistic approach to therapy, someone who understands the interconnectedness of your inner parts and can help you work towards balance and restoration.

   - **Support Groups**

     Support groups provide a space to share your story and connect with others who are navigating similar healing paths. Hearing others' journeys can offer insight, solidarity, and simple yet powerful solutions.

Guided Meditation: Merging the Fragments of Your Identity

This guided visualisation is designed to help you integrate the fragmented parts of yourself so you can reconnect with your whole and complete being.

1. **Preparation**

   Find a quiet, undisturbed space free from sensory distractions. Set aside 20 to 30 minutes. Sit or lie down comfortably. Close your eyes and prepare to listen and immerse yourself in the process.

2. **Settle In**

   Begin by settling into your chosen position. Close your eyes and take a few deep breaths. With each breath, allow your body to release tension. Let your muscles relax and your mind ease into a calm, composed, and centred state.

3. **Recognising Parts of Self**

   As you focus on your breath, bring awareness to every part of you that is seeking healing—your physical, emotional, mental, and spiritual selves. Visualise each part as its own distinct entity. Acknowledge and honour each one, recognising its place and importance in the totality of your being.

4. **Healing Light**

   Now, imagine a warm, healing light enveloping each part of yourself. Visualise this light as a nurturing energy that brings harmony and renewal. Allow this healing light to unite these parts, forming a single, cohesive whole.

5. **Empowerment Affirmations**

   Now, silently repeat the following affirmations with conviction and energy:

   - 'I am complete in all aspects.'
   - 'I am in unity with all emotions, which are parts of my being.'
   - 'Every piece of me is an essential part of the whole.'

6. **Transforming Inner Doubts**

   Continue with affirmations that dissolve any lingering doubt:

   - 'I am enough.'
   - 'All of me is healed.'
   - 'I am at peace with myself.'
   - 'I accept and appreciate every part of me.'
   - 'I am complete and centred.'

7. **Future Visualisation**

   Now, imagine yourself stepping into your future. See yourself embracing opportunities, overcoming challenges, and moving through life with clarity and confidence. Visualise yourself achieving your dreams and enjoying the life you desire. Know that the strength, peace, and empowerment you seek already exist within you.

8. **Closing**

   Take a few final deep breaths, this time breathing in a feeling of unity and wholeness. Let this feeling spread through your entire body. Slowly bring your awareness back to the present moment. Gently move your fingers and toes. Take a few more natural breaths, and when you are ready, open your eyes, feeling refreshed, whole, and in control of your life.

Case Study: From Fragmentation to Wholeness

Ravi, a client, presented with fragmented personalities and had previously been diagnosed with behavioural disorders. As noted earlier, fragmentation occurs when there is a dissociation between one's internal mental image of the world and the external reality. In Ravi's case, the fragmentation centred on an inability to assert himself—being consistently passive and never speaking up—until his suppressed emotions erupted in violent fits of rage.

When working with fragmentation, it is essential to recognise that these various selves are not pathological aberrations, but rather parts of the self left unnurtured due to life circumstances. For Ravi, early experiences of betrayal and bullying—particularly at the hands of close friends—had shaped a behavioural cycle of excessive meekness followed by explosive outbursts, a pattern that seemed to serve as a defence against perceived injustice and betrayal.

It was vital to acknowledge and engage with Ravi's child self, the part of him that most often interacted with the outside world. Through this self, it became clear that Ravi lived in a state of perpetual guardedness, always anticipating betrayal. This constant vigilance made it nearly impossible for him to let others into his inner world, straining his personal, social, and professional relationships. His hyperawareness kept him trapped in a loop of chronic stress, leaving him perpetually on edge and only one trigger away from an emotional eruption. These eruptions often escalated into sudden violent outbursts and, at times, physical altercations.

A critical step in therapy was validating his emotional responses. Ravi carried deep guilt over his past violent behaviour and felt frustrated and misunderstood when others dismissed his fears of being plotted against. While his hyperawareness and anticipation of betrayal undoubtedly coloured his perceptions, the emotional truth of his lived experiences could not be discounted. Acknowledging his subjective reality was vital, especially as he had likely encountered very few people who genuinely listened to or believed him. Within a space of acceptance, Ravi began to reveal more of his normal self, a part that existed in the middle ground between extreme passivity and explosive anger.

Therapy revealed that Ravi's passive self was rooted in a fear of conflict, while his violent self emerged from long-suppressed frustration erupting without regulation. Working within this framework, he gradually developed healthier coping mechanisms and learned to assert himself more constructively. He began finding ways to speak up and stand his ground without resorting to aggression. These new patterns transformed the way he engaged with the world. Slowly, his internal mental image began to align with his external reality, allowing the disparate parts of his self to integrate into a more cohesive whole.

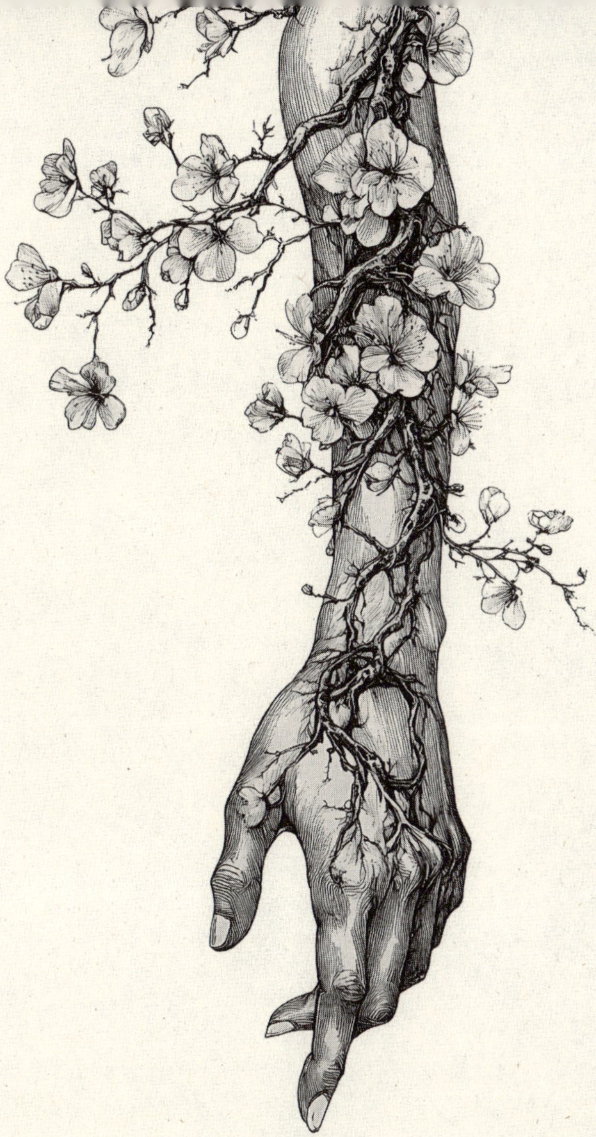

Part III

Transformation and Renewal

Chapter 10

The Healing PACT

'Trauma lives in the unspoken. Healing begins when we give it shape.'

The Nonlinear Nature of Healing

Healing is rarely a straight path. It doesn't unfold in neat, ascending stages or reward consistency with closure. Instead, it spirals, doubling back on itself, stalling unexpectedly, then surging forward with surprising clarity, only to pause again. Some days feel like progress and others feel like unravelling. Often, both happen in the same breath. This is not a flaw in the process. It is the process itself.

Unlike the narratives we are fed about 'getting over it' or 'moving on,' healing is not a finish line to be crossed. There is no final destination where we arrive unscarred, certain, or forever at peace. Rather, healing often reveals itself quietly, in small and tender moments that once felt out of reach—the pause instead of fleeing, the words spoken instead of silence, the softening instead of bracing. These are not grand gestures, but sacred ones. Markers not of perfection, but of change.

Yet many survivors of trauma, after doing the deep inner excavation—naming the wounds, tracing the patterns, finding the courage to remember, etc.—find themselves at a crossroads. They have insight. They have reclaimed their voice. Perhaps they have even offered forgiveness. But still, they ask: 'Now what?' and 'What comes after the naming, after the release?'

In such scenarios, what is often missing is not more knowledge but integration. Integration is the subtle yet essential process of weaving what we have learned into the way we live. It is what transforms insight into embodiment. It brings language into the body, awareness into the nervous system, and healing into the relational field, shaping how we connect with ourselves and with others in real time.

This phase of healing is rarely as dramatic as the breakthroughs that precede it. It is less about catharsis, more about cultivation and involves learning how to stay present with discomfort without drowning in it. It is practising new responses, over and over, even when they feel unnatural or vulnerable. It is noticing the small, hard-won shifts, like choosing rest without guilt, expressing a boundary without panic, or showing up as your full self without apology.

Integration isn't a checklist to be completed. It doesn't follow a timeline or a textbook. It moves more like a rhythm, i.e., something to be felt and followed, not forced. It is a lived, ongoing relationship with the self and a kind of inner pact. Put simply, it is a quiet commitment to show up, again and again, with compassion, curiosity, and care, especially on the days when the old patterns beckon or the progress feels invisible.

To integrate is to honour that healing is not only about what we survive but also about how we live after survival. It is about creating a life spacious enough to hold both pain and possibility. A life in which the past is acknowledged with tenderness but no longer dictates every choice. A life that makes room for the wounds without being wholly defined by them. This is the terrain of true transformation.

The Four-Part Awakening

Healing is often misunderstood as a single moment of breakthrough. People imagine it as the day you uncover the pattern, name the trauma, or finally connect the dots. But insight alone is not healing. You can know the cause, recite the triggers, even understand the timeline and still find yourself reacting in the same old ways.

True healing is a layered process. It doesn't begin the moment you discover the root. It begins when you allow yourself to stay with what you have found without fleeing, fixing, or folding. It requires presence, patience, and a kind of listening that goes deeper than logic.

This is where the PACT framework comes in: Presencing, Attunement, Curiosity, and Trust-Building. It is not a step-by-step guide, but a relational rhythm that can be returned to, cycled through, and lived with over time. It invites a slower, embodied kind of transformation. One that includes the nervous system, not just the mind. Let's explore this concept in great detail.

1. **Presencing: Regulate before You Reflect**

   Popularised in part by Otto Scharmer's work on Theory U at MIT, presencing combines the words 'presence and 'sensing,' referring to the ability to tune into and actualise emerging possibilities. In healing, it means arriving fully in your body before attempting to analyse your mind.

   For many survivors, insight comes faster than safety. They can explain everything but feel nothing. This is crucial as healing begins with safety in the body, not just intellectual understanding. That means slowing down, sensing the breath, feeling the ground, and noticing texture, tension, and tiny signals of aliveness. Put simply, presencing doesn't solve the problem but prepares you to meet it from a place of wholeness.

2. **Attunement: Listen beyond Language**

   Attunement is the capacity to listen deeply, not only to your thoughts or words but also to the subtle signals that lie beneath them. It is the moment you realise your 'yes' was actually a panic-fuelled nod, or that your endless productivity isn't motivation, but a shield against stillness.

   To be attuned is to notice the cues your body gives before the mind catches up. The shallow breath before people-pleasing. The jaw clench before setting a boundary. The withdrawal that hides a need for closeness. All in all, attunement helps us treat ourselves like living systems, not problems to solve.

3. **Curiosity: The Bridge from Reaction to Relationship**

   When healing turns into a performance—where we judge ourselves for every trigger or demand constant growth—we lose access to the gentler force of curiosity. And yet, curiosity is where self-compassion begins.

   Instead of labelling yourself as too much or not enough, curiosity invites you to ask: 'What might this reaction be trying to do for me?', 'What does this part of me need?', and 'What would happen if I approached this with wonder instead of war? This will help you slow down, stay present, and ground yourself more fully, creating a deeper sense of connection and stability.

4. **Trust-Building: Repair Happens in the Small Moments**

   Trust is often the slowest to return after trauma, especially the kind of trauma that made your own body or voice feel like the enemy. But it is also the most essential. Healing requires building trust with yourself, bit by bit, not through massive acts of self-love but through everyday choices.

   Rebuilding trust doesn't require grand gestures. It asks for consistency, honesty, and a willingness to choose yourself in micro-moments again and again.

In conclusion, it is important to remember that the PACT framework is not a rigid formula but a living rhythm. Presencing helps us arrive, attunement helps us listen, curiosity helps us understand, and trust helps us rebuild. These are not fixed stages but interconnected practices that you can return to in any order, at any time.

My hope is that you begin your journey of healing not as something to finish or achieve, but as an ongoing process that helps you deepen your connection with yourself, your story, and your innate capacity to begin again.

Chapter 11
Healing through Fiction

'Healing doesn't ask for proof. It asks for presence.'

The Use of Imagination in Healing

A common facet of therapy is the use of fiction when exploring one's inner world. This refers to the use of illusion, fantasy, or projection when expressing emotions or recounting trauma. Functioning as an extension of the inner child, it offers a way for individuals to maintain a connection with their childlike wonder, allowing them to make sense of the world while holding onto hope and dreams. This imaginative process naturally leads us to storytelling, a practice that not only entertains but also serves as a vital tool for emotional exploration and healing.

Storytelling is a unique activity that goes beyond mere entertainment. It is a powerful means of evoking and examining emotions, reshaping experiences, and fostering personal growth. In this sense, stories are not just accounts of our lives; they are the forces that shape and define our beliefs, behaviours, and identities. To meaningfully incorporate narrative strategies into therapy, it is important to examine what can be considered a narrative, what issues narratives can cause, and how certain stories may be rewritten in healing ways. This conscious rewriting allows us to release limiting patterns and create new meanings that support healing and transformation. Ultimately, the power of storytelling lies in its ability to reconnect us with our authentic selves, opening pathways toward greater resilience, understanding, and hope.

In this chapter, we will explore the profound influence that stories have on our lives, how they shape our sense of self, and their potential as powerful tools for transformation and healing. We will also examine the ways in which narratives can both limit and liberate us, and how conscious storytelling can become a catalyst for personal growth and renewed meaning.

The Power of Personal Narratives

The stories we tell ourselves influence how we see our identity and how we engage with the world. Recognising the power of storytelling in shaping our identity, behaviour, and emotions opens the door to transformation. By consciously reshaping these stories, we can rewrite our internal scripts and create new pathways toward healing and growth.

1. **Shaping Identity and Perception**
   Stories, especially those that are spoken or repeatedly internalised, can have a profound impact on the formation of one's identity and worldview. When internalised, certain narratives may cause individuals to highlight only the negative aspects of themselves or reinforce limiting beliefs about what they can achieve. For instance, someone who constantly tells themselves they are a failure or worthless is likely to develop low self-esteem and diminished self-worth.

2. **Reinforcing Patterns of Behaviour**

   Personal histories and internal narratives can also reinforce patterns of behaviour by solidifying certain self-concepts. For example, someone who believes they are the unluckiest person in the world may, often unconsciously, act in ways that validate this belief, turning it into a self-fulfilling prophecy.

3. **Taking Control of Emotional Experiences**

   While fiction can provide catharsis and aid in healing, it may also trap someone in a loop of unresolved emotion. For example, repeatedly telling a charged, emotionally heavy story without resolution can lead to self-victimisation rather than progress. Instead of moving through the pain, the person may remain emotionally stuck in that narrative.

Transformative Change via Storytelling

The following approaches offer practical ways to harness the potential of storytelling for healing and personal growth.

1. **Narrative Reframing**

   In mainstream therapy, narrative therapy frequently employs the technique of reframing. When individuals collaborate with therapists to retell their stories, they begin to:

   - **Externalise Problems:** They separate themselves from the problem, viewing it as something external rather than an inherent part of their identity.

- **Reauthor Their Stories:** They reframe their biographical narrative in ways that emphasise strengths, adaptability, resilience, and future possibilities, rather than dwelling on past failures and suffering.

2. **Building Self-Empowering Stories**

   Stories that foster self-empowerment focus on:

   - **Situational Strengths and Resilience:** Moments when the individual was courageous, showed maturity, or overcame significant challenges.
   - **Time Orientation:** A forward-looking mindset that embraces positive change and new possibilities.

3. **Changing Cognitions and Behaviour**

   To support narrative change, the following approaches may be used:

   - **Cognitive Restructuring:** Shifting focus from unhelpful beliefs to more constructive ones in order to influence behaviour positively.
   - **Behavioural Activation:** Taking deliberate action in line with the new, empowering narrative to reinforce meaningful change.

Guided Meditation: Changing the Life Story

This guided meditation is designed to help you shift your inner narratives in order to heal, to recover from crises, and to evolve as a more whole version of yourself.

1. **Preparation**

   Find a quiet and comfortable space where you won't be disturbed. You can choose to sit upright or lie down in a relaxed position. Gently close your eyes and take a few deep breaths, inhaling and exhaling slowly and mindfully.

2. **Grounding and Relaxation**

   Begin by bringing your full attention to your breath. Inhale deeply through your nose, allowing your lungs to fill fully, and then exhale slowly through your mouth. With each exhale, imagine releasing any tension or stress you are holding. Visualise each breath out as a cleansing wave, carrying away negative thoughts, self-doubt, and limiting beliefs. Let each exhale be a quiet act of release.

3. **Visualisation of the Current Narrative**

   Now, bring to mind the story or narrative that seems to define your current life. It might be a story of hardship, limitations, or failure. See this narrative clearly by visualising it like a scene in a film or a page in a book. Make it as vivid as you can.

4. **Identifying Limiting Beliefs**

   Within this story, gently identify the beliefs, assumptions, or repeated messages that are troubling or holding you back, whether logically or emotionally. Acknowledge these beliefs without judgement. Allow them to be there, simply observing their presence and influence.

5. **Exteriorisation and Projection**

   Now, begin to imagine this story as something external to you. See it as being projected outward, as if it belongs to a character separate from you. Visualise how this narrative has shaped your thoughts, your emotions, and your actions. Witness it from a slight distance, with compassion and curiosity.

6. **Redrawing the Story**

   At this point, imagine that you are holding the pen. You have the power to revise this narrative. Begin to rewrite the story in a way that aligns with healing, strength, and possibility. Reconstruct the moments, reframe the meanings, and add new chapters that reflect resilience, growth, and clarity. Allow yourself to author a version of the story where you are no longer stuck in past patterns but are moving forward with purpose and self-trust.

Case Study: Balancing the Rational Mind with the Emotional Self

Within therapy sessions, clients and therapists often engage in psychodrama, which is a technique where the client dramatically interacts with various aspects of themselves. This process enables deeper emotional processing and fosters greater awareness of their emotions and attachment styles. Clients who engage in psychodrama commonly report enhanced self-confidence, improved relationships, strengthened listening skills and empathy, healthier coping mechanisms, and a renewed sense of hope. Dramatic engagement is also linked to greater in-session cognitive and emotional exploration, more significant therapeutic breakthroughs, and reduced resistance to change.

Therapists often use a combination of cognitive-behavioural and narrative techniques to encourage this process. The goal is to access different facets of the self and weave them into a more coherent, integrated whole while also nurturing a sense of possibility and hope.

The following case illustrates how one client used storytelling, fantasy, and projection to engage with difficult emotions and concepts.

Client Rohan presented with a sense of being stuck, blocked from growth and unable to move towards meaningful change. Over the course of therapy, it became evident that Rohan had a strong tendency to interpret everything through a strictly rational lens. He deeply believed that intellectual ability and reasoning were central to making sense of the world and deriving meaning from it.

In contrast, another client, Aditya, viewed intellect as a means of proving their worth to both their parents and society. For them, academic excellence was evidence of their perseverance and a way of rising above their circumstances and inner struggles.

It is essential to understand that clients who show resistance to therapy—especially when it involves non-traditional or experiential techniques—often over-identify with their rational and intellectual selves. This overemphasis can serve as a way of declaring their disbelief in anything not deemed 'scientific,' making it clear that they do not subscribe to therapeutic approaches they view as vague or intangible.

Working with such clients requires engaging with them from within their own narrative and framework. People tend to feel in control when they operate within this rational space, and the fear of the unknown—or anything beyond that space—often keeps them firmly rooted there. They equate control with freedom and are deeply uncomfortable with the idea of surrendering to unpredictable or uncontrollable elements that may bring change.

In such cases, therapy centres on creating a safe, supportive environment where the client can gradually feel secure enough to be vulnerable. Clients are encouraged to reflect on their life experiences and articulate their emotions in ways that allow them to recognise logical patterns in their thoughts and behaviours. As their comfort with emotional expression grows, the therapy can transition into a more gestalt-based approach. Techniques such as projection and emotional externalisation—like the empty chair exercise—are introduced, allowing clients to revisit and process experiences that fall outside their existing worldview or logical framework. Gestalt work helps such clients slowly develop psychological flexibility and a greater sense of agency when faced with unfamiliar or emotionally confusing situations. Over time, they learn healthier and more constructive ways of responding to these experiences.

Another important consideration when working with highly rational clients is their tendency to overthink and ruminate. They often become stuck in cognitive loops, replaying specific events repeatedly. This habit can interfere with therapy, as it distracts them from the present moment and the therapeutic work at hand.

To address this, person-centred and gestalt approaches employ a variety of techniques, including immediate feedback, reflecting both content and emotion, paraphrasing, summarising, slowing the session down to delve deeper into key areas, and using immediacy to gently bring the client back to the present. A simple yet effective technique is to reframe past events in the present tense by asking the client how they feel now about something they are recalling from the past. Often, their emotional response changes when asked to express their present experience rather than simply narrate the past.

A final and often critical area of work with such clients involves creative self-expression. Earlier theories—like those of Freud—saw creativity as a socially acceptable outlet for inner desires. More recent perspectives, such as those from Rogers and Eysenck, view creativity as a reflection of individual uniqueness and a key driver of self-development and self-actualisation.

Importantly, creativity thrives on intrinsic motivation and a non-judgemental mindset. When expression is externally controlled or evaluated, it limits authenticity and suppresses the natural creative process. Clients who are highly focused on logic often disconnect from this expressive side of themselves, possibly because creativity doesn't follow fixed rules or a defined structure. It is fluid, emotional, and at times, even chaotic. Such qualities can feel threatening to the logical mind.

Creativity arises from the interaction between cognitive processes, personality traits, emotional patterns, and one's environment. For individuals who prioritise rationality, embracing this unpredictable and emotive form of expression can be daunting. Thus, therapy with such clients not only supports healthy emotional exploration but also gently guides them towards experiencing the freedom and personal growth that comes from authentic creative expression.

Chapter 12

Barriers to Healing

'Barriers to healing often arise not from what blocks us, but from what we have yet to understand within ourselves.'

There are many factors that can hinder the therapeutic process and become barriers in an individual's healing journey. Recognising these barriers becomes extremely important when working with clients, so as to be able to dissolve them and open up the path for change and growth to take place.

One of the most common and deeply ingrained of these barriers is the body's habitual stress response. Stress stimulates a reaction known as the fight–flight–or–freeze response in the body, which involves physiological arousal and a release of stress hormones such as cortisol and adrenaline. We become so accustomed to reacting in these ways to life situations that these reactions themselves start acting as barriers to healing. Healing, on the other hand, requires a different kind of response, and this can feel very uncomfortable for people because it brings up the very feelings they have been suppressing. The therapist supports and gently handholds them through the process of facing these situations in a new way.

To support this shift, therapeutic approaches that calm the nervous system and gently rewire conditioned responses become essential. In the following sections, we explore methods that help restore the mind and body to a state of balance and openness to healing.

Subconscious Oaths and Vows

Subconscious oaths operate as deep-rooted programs within the subconscious mind. They influence how we think, feel, act, and even how we form or sustain healthy relationships. These internalised vows often remain hidden from our conscious awareness, yet they shape our choices, reactions, and patterns in life. Whether related to love, trust, success, or self-worth, such oaths can create invisible boundaries that govern how we engage with the world.

As Okken states, 'Promises make debts.' What this suggests is that people often make subconscious oaths and vows in emotionally intense moments. For instance, after experiencing heartbreak, one might vow to never love again. Or after witnessing dysfunctional relationships in childhood, one might quietly decide that it is not worth bringing a child into such a world. These are powerful, emotionally charged vows made in response to deep pain, and they can become more binding than we consciously realise.

Even seemingly innocent promises made during childhood—such as pledging to always be honest, loyal, or kind—can become long-standing internal rules. As the idealism of childhood meets the complexity of adult life, the reality of a less-than-perfect world can create inner conflict. People struggle to live up to those vows and, when they can't, experience guilt, frustration, or a sense of personal betrayal towards themselves, their parents or guardians, or even their understanding of God.

Often, these vows are buried so deeply in the subconscious that they manifest as patterns or life experiences that feel puzzling or overwhelming. Working with such subconscious oaths usually begins with recognising them, which is often the hardest step.

In the next section, we will examine how these subconscious beliefs, oaths, and vows manifest in our lives and the effects they can have on our thoughts, behaviours, and overall well-being.

How Subconscious Beliefs and Inner Vows Shape Us

As discussed, our subconscious beliefs and inner vows often operate beneath the surface, quietly influencing our identity, choices, and patterns. Let's take a closer look at some of the key ways in which these subconscious beliefs and inner vows shape our lives, often influencing us more than we realise.

1. **Guiding Behaviour and Choices**

   Subconscious beliefs do not lie dormant in a person's mind. They actively guide behaviour and decision-making, especially in areas related to health, relationships, and self-care practices.

2. **Impact on Health**

   Negative subconscious beliefs—such as persistent feelings of worthlessness, deep grief, or unresolved emotional pain—can sometimes give rise to destructive desires, including self-sabotage or self-annihilation. These internal conflicts may manifest in physical conditions like autoimmune disorders.

3. **Pattern Formation**

   These beliefs often act like magnets, drawing repetitive cycles of self-destruction, limitation, or disempowerment. Over time, they can deteriorate overall well-being and life quality. They get activated automatically in response to life events, manifesting as recurring abusive relationships, frequent accidents, or chronic illness.

Methods of Reconditioning the Mind Back to Its Original State

Transforming subconscious beliefs requires not just awareness but deliberate and consistent practice. The following steps outline practical methods that support this inner work, each offering a way to access, understand, and reshape the beliefs that silently shape our lives.

1. **Self-Cognisance and Its Effective Practice Systems**

   Self-cognisance—combined with reflective practices such as journaling—helps reveal deep-seated subconscious beliefs and behavioural patterns. Observing these thought processes, emotions, and recurring life issues helps in identifying underlying beliefs that may be impacting one's health and overall well-being.

2. **Use of Affirmations**

   Positive affirmations can be effective tools in transforming destructive subconscious belief systems. By consistently repeating affirmations that focus on health, well-being, and self-worth, individuals begin to gradually reprogram the subconscious mind towards more empowering beliefs.

3. **Hypnosis and Visualisation**

   Both hypnosis and visualisation work because the subconscious mind is highly receptive to suggestion. Through deep relaxation and guided imagery, individuals can access stored beliefs and introduce constructive, healing suggestions to support change.

Guided Meditation: Letting Go of Subconscious Oaths

Guided meditation creates a calm, focused state in which the subconscious mind becomes more accessible and open to change. Through intentional visualisation and gentle suggestion, individuals can identify old inner vows and release them with greater ease. This process allows for emotional healing, creating space for new, empowering beliefs to take root. Over time, it supports a sense of inner freedom and clarity.

Given below is a step-by-step guided meditation to help you let go of subconscious oaths and open yourself to renewed possibilities.

1. **Preparation**

   Choose a clean, quiet space where you won't be disturbed. Sit or recline in a comfortable position, allowing your muscles to relax. Close your eyes and begin taking slow, deep breaths, gradually calming your mind and allowing your body to soften and settle.

2. **Entering a State of Relaxation**

   Imagine yourself standing at the top of a staircase that leads into a deeper space within your subconscious mind. Visualise the stairs stretching downward in front of you. With each step you take, allow any tension within you to gently melt away, and feel your connection with your innermost self deepen.

3. **Entering the Subconscious**

   As you reach the final step, see yourself standing in a still, secure space within your mind. This space represents an active part of your inner world—the subconscious—where your most deeply held beliefs are stored and can now be gently explored.

4. **Discovering Buried Vows**

   Let yourself be wrapped in a sense of calm and peace in this space. Now ask your inner self to reveal any oaths, vows, or pledges you may have taken, whether in this lifetime or another. Allow them to come into your awareness without resistance, judgement, or fear. Simply observe what arises.

5. **Letting Go of the Oaths Symbolically**

   Now begin to visualise these oaths and vows as symbols or images in your mind's eye. Invite a gentle healing light to flow into this space. Watch as the light envelops each image, softly dissolving them and releasing their hold on your subconscious.

6. **Closing and Affirmation**

   Either silently or aloud, repeat the following affirmation: 'All oaths I have made that no longer serve me are now null and void. I am at peace in my body. I choose love, health, and self-empowerment.' Allow yourself to fully feel the soothing and empowering energy of this affirmation as it becomes a part of your being.

7. **Grounding**

   Remain still for a moment and enjoy the peaceful sensation of having released these subconscious bonds. When you are ready, begin to return to the present moment in whatever way feels right for you. Gently move your fingers and toes, stretch your body, and when it feels natural, open your eyes. You are now grounded, free, and renewed.

Case Study: Invisible Bonds and Restraints

Anita presented with ongoing feelings of sadness and frustration and reported difficulties in nearly all of her personal relationships. Her spouse, Arjun, was also undergoing therapy.

Anita described challenges not only with her spouse but also with her in-laws, her mother, her sibling, and even within herself, as she constantly suppressed her own anger and emotional needs. She found her spouse to be argumentative and prone to conflict, while her in-laws were perceived as unsupportive and emotionally distant. In response, she tended to hold back emotional expression in order to avoid triggering arguments or discomfort.

Additionally, Anita's parents frequently appeared helpless and in need of support. She experienced intense guilt over having moved out and leaving them behind. Financial stress was another factor, as she felt restricted around money and feared being judged by her spouse for her financial decisions.

On the other hand, Arjun did not believe that any major incident had occurred to explain why Anita felt so emotionally constrained. He suggested that her difficulty in setting boundaries with her parents may have been a key contributing factor, noting that Anita often struggled to say no or assert her needs.

There also appeared to be a connection between Anita's childhood experiences and the challenges she faced in the present. Beyond the difficulties in various relationships, her tendency to suppress herself, her recurring guilt over not being available to loved ones, and her fear of being judged seemed to stem from formative experiences during her early years.

The concept of the abandoned or orphaned inner child—in which a child feels emotionally rejected or left behind and is forced to become their own parent—emerged as significant in Anita's case. Moreover, having lost one parent early in life, she assumed a parental role within the family, effectively missing out on a full experience of her own childhood. During adolescence, she recalled being the one who held the family together following the passing of her second parent. She described this role as a burden, often acting as a parent to her younger sibling while simultaneously being reprimanded by relatives for doing so. This contradiction created a deep sense of resentment, as she was blamed while trying to do what felt right. Phrases like 'be quiet' were frequently used, and these experiences were linked to her current difficulty in expressing emotions or voicing concerns.

The internal conflict between being an elder sibling and taking on a parental role remained unresolved and continued to impact Anita's life. During therapy, this tension was explored. A discussion was initiated about the importance of respecting others' space, boundaries, and agency. To support emotional release, guided imagery was introduced, in which Anita visualised her family members in the room. Techniques such as projection and externalisation were used to help her symbolically relinquish these burdensome roles and return them to their original source: her parents.

At the same time, Anita was guided to reclaim her rightful place as the child within the family system. This emotional unburdening was seen as a crucial first step towards reconnecting with her inner child and beginning to experience life with greater freedom and authenticity. As part of this process, Anita participated in an empty chair exercise, in which she spoke openly to her family members, expressing her true thoughts and feelings.

A follow-up guided imagery session involved Anita's spouse and in-laws. Anita described her in-laws as perfectionistic and expressed a belief that Arjun harboured a fear of punishment. Arjun acknowledged that while his parents were not overtly controlling, they tended to comply with their own parents' wishes out of habit or respect.

At this stage, the focus shifted to how subconscious familial bonds and unresolved emotional burdens were affecting the couple's relationship. A discussion followed, exploring how both Anita and Arjun were caught in patterns centred on pleasing others, which prevented them from forming a deeper emotional connection. Releasing these subconscious ties was seen as essential for shifting focus back towards themselves and their relationship. They were encouraged to nurture their bond and prioritise self-care alongside their commitment to each other.

In conclusion, Anita's journey in therapy reflected the unravelling of long-standing emotional patterns rooted in family dynamics, loss, and internalised expectations. Through a blend of emotional processing and therapeutic techniques, she began the process of letting go of burdens that were never truly hers to carry. The hope moving forward lay in Anita and Arjun choosing to build a relationship anchored in self-awareness, compassion, and shared emotional responsibility.

Chapter 13
Healing Beyond the Session

'Lasting change happens when healing becomes a practice, not just a process.'

Living the Healing Process

HEALING IS A NATURAL PROCESS THAT UNFOLDS WHEN a client is provided a safe and non-judgemental space. A space where the client can voice suppressed feelings without slipping into guilt. After the catharsis of a therapy session, the client returns to their everyday life. While no one around them has changed, the client begins to see and feel a difference in their body, their relationships, and their overall experience of life.

This emerging awareness often unfolds gradually, sometimes in subtle shifts rather than dramatic moments. It is in these everyday experiences that the seeds of transformation take root. This is when the client realises that the real battles were never outside; they were always within. They begin to recognise how constantly they were creating their reality based on assumptions of what might happen and reacting from that place. But none of that was ever the real problem. Each problem was, in fact, an opportunity for self-exploration and a chance to shift one's thought process. And this understanding marks a profound shift in the client's inner world. They begin to move out of blame, shame, guilt, and regret. Life starts to be lived from a space of choice and possibility, and they begin to take charge, rather than trying to control life and people out of fear.

Healing beyond the session is an ongoing journey—a continuous unfolding of insight, acceptance, and growth that extends far beyond the therapist's office. It calls for patience, self-compassion, and courage to face the unknown within. Ultimately, it invites the client to become an active participant in their own transformation, embodying the changes and integrating them into daily life, thus turning healing into a lived reality.

Healing as a Network

As discussed in the previous sections, what happens within the therapeutic space is often only a fraction of the healing that actually takes place. A significant amount of progress occurs outside the therapist's office, and this healing frequently extends to the client's friends and family as well.

In some cases, people from the client's life may begin seeking therapy themselves. In other instances, individuals around the client experience healing indirectly through the client's journey. The threads that connect us—the bonds between people—often function as channels through which healing flows, back and forth. Jungian psychology calls this shared resonance the collective unconscious, which is a system of symbolic meanings carrying both personal significance and broader collective meaning. In essence, when one person heals, that healing often reaches beyond the individual to touch a group, a community, or even an entire network.

This interconnected nature of healing reminds us that personal transformation is never isolated. Each step forward ripples outward, influencing relationships, communities, and the larger social fabric. Embracing healing as a network not only honours the complexity of human connection but also invites us to participate in a shared journey toward wholeness and collective well-being.

Case Study: Mutual Healing and Support

Samar came into therapy presenting with stress related to professional responsibilities. He was accompanied by his parent, Lalit, who came as moral support. While Samar attended his session, Lalit chose to speak with another therapist.

Lalit presented with feelings of hopelessness and a lack of motivation or desire. Having spent a lifetime cycling through multiple roles—spouse, parent, engineer, and teacher—Lalit was now retired. His spouse had passed away, and his children were settled with families of their own. At this stage, Lalit seemed to believe that he had lived his life, and there was nothing meaningful left to look forward to.

As the conversation deepened, it became clear that Lalit was grieving, not just the loss of his spouse, but also the loss of identity that had once come from being the head of the school he had founded. He appeared resigned to a life of quiet sadness, not seeing the possibility of a vibrant or fulfilling old age. Hobbies and interests were spoken of as distant ifs, not real, accessible pursuits.

Lalit described his time as an engineer as both rewarding and draining. He had been passionate about the work, yet often felt like a mule: going to work, toiling endlessly, returning home, raising children, and repeating the cycle. The experience had left him stressed and unfulfilled.

Interestingly, in his own session, Samar echoed a strikingly similar description of his life. Both saw reflections of themselves in the other, offering a powerful insight into the generational patterns and emotional resonance shared between family members.

After leaving engineering, Lalit had gone on to open a school, which had given him a renewed sense of purpose and a way to give back to the community. He had hoped that Samar would find a similar channel—something meaningful that could help him release his stress. Meanwhile, Samar described a range of passions and hobbies he enjoyed and expressed a wish for Lalit to rediscover his own zest for life and begin living more fully again. Despite the age and context differences, both had navigated similar stressors and had held within them perspectives and wisdom that could deeply support one another.

In the days following their sessions, Lalit shared that he had indeed begun rediscovering small joys and had started showing early signs of embracing life again. Samar, too, had gradually begun coping with stress in far healthier ways.

Chapter 14

Healing the Healer

'To heal others deeply, the healer must first tend to their own inner landscape with equal care.'

Working with Medical and Mental Health Professionals

THOSE IN HEALING PROFESSIONS—THERAPISTS, DOCTORS, nurses, and social workers—often face emotionally intense and high-pressure environments. Over time, this can lead to burnout, compassion fatigue, and chronic stress. People in such roles frequently prioritise their patients' and clients' well-being over their own. Yet, self-care and creating space for one's own healing are essential, especially because these professions can be physically, mentally, and emotionally depleting.

For instance, when doctors fall ill themselves, they may experience guilt or frustration over not being able to continue their work, often internalising this as being a bad doctor or even a bad person. Yet caring for others should never come at the expense of caring for oneself. By tending to their own needs—through rest, therapy, spiritual practice, or quiet reflection—healers protect their health while renewing the energy, empathy, and clarity they bring to their work. In doing so, they model healthy boundaries and self-compassion, showing that true service is sustained not by relentless self-sacrifice, but by a balanced, replenished self. This balance between self-care and caregiving is essential for their mental and emotional well-being.

Healing the Self

People in healing professions and those in other helping roles, like teaching or the clergy, often operate in highly demanding and emotionally taxing spaces. They frequently report suffering from emotional and compassion fatigue, burnout, and stress. It is an unfortunate aspect of the helper's role that they often devote far more energy to serving others than they do to caring for themselves. Additionally, individuals in these fields are often highly self-critical about their contributions to others' lives, grappling with self-doubt, fear of failure, and a diminished sense of confidence when they feel they have been unable to help someone.

Learning appropriate self-care is an area frequently overlooked in helping professions. However, when this is neglected, it eventually renders them incapable of continuing their work effectively. Only a person who feels physically, emotionally, and mentally well can truly offer help to others without absorbing their distress or succumbing to secondary stress. When caregivers ignore their own needs while continuing to support others, they often reach a point of mental, emotional, and physical exhaustion and may ultimately require care themselves.

Striking a balance between caring for yourself and caring for others is an essential lesson for everyone, not only for those in helping professions. Both the personal and professional self must be nurtured and kept in equilibrium for a person to feel whole and at peace. The path to achieving this balance involves compassion towards oneself, the practice of self-love and forgiveness, and a deep commitment to introspection.

There are several self-care strategies individuals can incorporate, including creating a self-care action plan, using self-care checklists, seeking therapy or support when needed, and leaning on family and friends for support. Other methods include self-assessments, journaling, and engaging in activities that promote rest and renewal.

By making self-care a non-negotiable part of daily life, helpers safeguard their ability to show up fully, with clarity, patience, and presence. This ongoing investment in one's own well-being not only prevents burnout but also allows the act of helping to remain a source of joy and purpose, rather than depletion.

Learning to Heal the Healers

Learning to heal the healers is crucial, whether you are a student of psychology, a practicing therapist, or even a homemaker. Healers, including therapists, doctors, and caregivers, are central to the healing process, and their well-being directly impacts the quality of care they provide. Even if you are not formally in a healing profession, you are constantly healing in your own way, comforting loved ones, easing the pain of others if you are an empath, or, if you are a spiritual empath, sensing a deep connection with all beings and carrying a desire to alleviate suffering from the world.

When healers become emotionally or mentally exhausted, they may struggle to provide the empathy, insight, and presence that their clients need for meaningful recovery. In contrast, healers who prioritise their own self-care are better equipped to create a safe, compassionate space, which in turn leads to deeper, more effective healing for others.

Moreover, when clients understand that healers, too, need care, it humanises the relationship. This realisation fosters mutual respect and trust and encourages clients to take a more active role in their own healing journey. A healthy, balanced healer is more capable of offering thoughtful, attuned guidance, often inspiring clients to fully commit to their process of healing.

In the larger picture, nurturing the healer is not just about sustaining one individual; it is about preserving the integrity of the entire healing process. Every act of self-renewal a healer undertakes ripples outward, strengthening the web of care that binds communities together. By honouring their own limits, celebrating their own humanity, and engaging in practices that restore their mind, body, and spirit, healers embody the truth that healing is a shared journey that thrives when both giver and receiver are nourished.

Strategies and Resources for Healer Self-Care

Healers can support their own well-being through practices like meditation, consulting with supervisors, participating in supportive peer networks, and engaging in ongoing professional development. These approaches help reduce stress, prevent burnout, and support the continual growth of the self.

1. **Prioritise Self-Care**

   Make self-care a non-negotiable part of your life. Regardless of cultural expectations or external responsibilities, caregivers must engage in nurturing practices that support the mind, body, and spirit.

2. **Seek Supervision and Support**

   It is essential to participate in regular supervision and peer support groups. These spaces allow caregivers to share experiences, gain insight, and receive emotional reinforcement from those who understand the demands of the work.

3. **Engage in Continuous Professional Development**

   Staying updated through ongoing professional development can play a key role in preventing burnout. While research varies, many studies suggest that learning new tools and expanding one's perspective can help caregivers cope with work-related stress and remain engaged in their roles.

Guided Self-Meditation: Self-Care for Healers

This guided meditation is designed to help you cultivate a deep sense of self-care and nurturing. By inviting your mind and body into a peaceful, safe space, you can reconnect with your inner well-being and foster healing from within. Follow the steps below to gently soothe yourself and reinforce the intention of care and restoration.

1. **Preparation**

   Sit or lie down in a position that feels natural and relaxed. Close your eyes. Take a few deep breaths, gently letting your body know it is safe to soften and unwind.

2. **Visualise Self-Care**

   Picture yourself in a space that brings you peace and calm, perhaps a serene garden, a cosy room, or a rejuvenating spa. Let your mind settle into this place.

3. **Imagine Self-Nurturing Activities**

   In this setting, visualise yourself engaging in soothing and nourishing activities, like soaking in a warm bath, receiving a gentle massage, or simply sitting in quiet meditation.

4. **Affirmations**

   As you relax into this imagery, gently repeat affirmations such as:

   - 'I take care of myself.'
   - 'I am held, and I am healed.'
   - 'I am healing, and I am whole.'

5. **Closing the Practice**

   In Indian philosophy, a simple guiding phrase is: 'Inhale strength, exhale weakness.' Take a few more deep breaths, feeling replenished. Slowly bring your awareness back to the room. When you feel ready, open your eyes, carrying this sense of care with you.

Case Study: Trauma and Intimacy

Sakshi presented with difficulty in social situations, particularly in interacting comfortably within groups. She identified as introverted and reported challenges with emotional and physical intimacy.

Sakshi was visibly uneasy with discussions around intimacy. As therapy progressed, it became evident that this discomfort could be traced back to a childhood experience where she had witnessed physical intimacy between her parents. As a child, Sakshi had misinterpreted the act, believing her mother was in pain. As a result, she had formed an early association between intimacy, pain, and rejection. These experiences had left her feeling unloved and pushed aside, prompting a desire to emotionally withdraw.

Freud noted that children often try to emulate the parent of the same gender and seek partners who resemble the opposite-sex parent. When children witness intimacy between their parents, it can evoke feelings of exclusion or emotional rejection. In Sakshi's case, this dynamic had reinforced the belief that love meant being replaced or becoming secondary, especially to her father's affections. This early emotional injury had deeply affected Sakshi's ability to connect and feel safe in intimate relationships later in life.

Therapy for Sakshi focused on unpacking her perceptions of love and intimacy. Narrative therapy and storytelling were chosen as the primary interventions, as she naturally leaned towards expressing herself through personal narratives. These approaches had allowed Sakshi to explore her internalised stories and begin reshaping them.

Cognitive restructuring was used to help Sakshi reframe her past experiences, transforming the narrative that love and intimacy must involve physical pain or rejection. Visualisation techniques had helped her perceive love and intimacy as multi-layered experiences that could be nurturing and safe, rather than painful or threatening. Through these exercises, intimacy was redefined as a complex and nuanced form of connection. It was no longer seen as solely or necessarily physical, and it was certainly not confused with harm.

An interesting therapeutic insight emerged when examining Sakshi's professional life. She worked in emergency services, frequently exposed to traumatic situations. This may not have been coincidental. Often, people are drawn to environments that mirror unresolved inner experiences. In Sakshi's case, working in trauma settings might have served as a way to vicariously confront and process her own buried pain.

Gestalt theory describes projection as a defence mechanism by which individuals unconsciously externalise parts of themselves they find difficult to face. These aspects then attach to external situations or people. This mechanism can offer a less threatening path to healing, allowing the person to examine painful emotions or past events indirectly, at a safe psychological distance. For Sakshi, this therapeutic insight had opened a door towards understanding her own emotional patterns and how her professional environment might have been providing an unexpected space for inner resolution.

Acknowledgements

No journey is ever travelled alone, and I owe much of mine to the people who have stood beside me with patience and love.

This book would not exist without the quiet strength, unconditional support, and infinite patience of my family, especially my parents, whose wisdom has been my compass, and my teacher, who has always believed in the healing power of words.

I would also like to express my gratitude to the many people who shared their most vulnerable stories with me. Your honesty, courage, and trust have shaped every page. You are the true teachers of this work.

My heartfelt thanks to the entire team at Hay House for believing in the vision of this book. In particular, I am indebted to Aditya Jarial, whose thoughtful editing, encouragement, and gentle yet firm deadlines helped me refine my voice and bring clarity to my message. You gave this book not just structure but also soul.

I am equally grateful to my mentors, fellow healers, and friends, whose insights into the human mind, body, and spirit have enriched my understanding of emotional and physical well-being. Thank you for the late-night conversations, the challenges that helped me grow, and the laughter that reminded me to stay grounded.

A special note of gratitude to my friends, both old and new, who kept me inspired, nourished, and joyful throughout the long months of writing. You are my anchors and my cheerleaders.

And finally, I wish to thank every reader who picks up this book. May you find in these pages a mirror for your own emotions, a deeper connection with your body, and the courage to heal from the inside out.

References

1. Ahlin, E. M. (2013). *Youth involvement in crime: The importance of locus of control and collective efficacy*. Retrieved from https://ebookcentral.proquest.com/lib/acap/detail.action?docID=1057785.

2. Allan, C. (2006). In the room: Case conceptualisation I. Retrieved April 29, 2011, from http://gandalwaven.typepad.com/intheroom/2006/09/case_conceptual.html.

3. Avest, I. (2017). "I experienced freedom within the frame of my own narrative": The contribution of psychodrama techniques to experiential learning in teacher training. *International Review of Education, 63*(1), 71–86.

4. Azoulay, B., & Orkibi, H. (2015). The four-phase CBN psychodrama model: A manualised approach for practice and research. *The Arts in Psychotherapy, 42*, 10–18. https://doi.org/10.1016/j.aip.2014.12.012.

5. Banmen, J. (1982). The use of humour in psychotherapy. *International Journal for the Advancement of Counselling, 5*(2), 81–86.

6. Barnett, B. (2007). *You ought to!: A psychoanalytic study of the superego and conscience*. Retrieved from https://ebookcentral.proquest.com.

7. Beaumont, A. (2015, September 11). Fat is an emotional issue. Retrieved November 12, 2017, from https://www.psychologytoday.com/blog/handy-hints-humans/201509/fat-is-emotional-issue.

8. Benjamin, J. (2013, October 17). Sometimes (I'm schizoaffective) / All of the time (I'm human). Retrieved from https://www.youtube.com/watch?v=M3_hny4GFlY.

9. Bloch, A. (Director), & Bloch, A. (Producer). (2006). *The mind-body connection* [Video file]. Thinking Allowed Productions. Retrieved from Counseling and Therapy in Video: Classic database.

10. Bowlby, J. (1969/1982). *Attachment and loss. Vol. 1: Attachment.* New York: Basic Books.

11. Chowdhary, S., & Gopinath, J. (2013). Clinical hypnosis and Patanjali yoga sutras. *Indian Journal of Psychiatry, 55*, 157–164.

12. Clear, J. (2017, September 26). How long does it actually take to form a new habit? Backed by science. Retrieved November 18, 2017, from https://jamesclear.com/new-habit.

13. Crago, H., & Gardner, P. (2012). Being there: Developing the capacity for holding. In *A safe place for change* (pp. 20–49). Melbourne, Australia: IP Communications.

14. Dakis, J., & Singh, B. S. (1994). Making sense of the psychiatric patient. In B. S. Bloch & B. S. Singh (Eds.), *Foundations of clinical psychiatry*. Melbourne: Melbourne University Press.

15. Dogan, T. (2010). The effects of psychodrama on young adults' attachment styles. *The Arts in Psychotherapy, 37*(2), 112–119. https://doi.org/10.1016/j.aip.2010.02.001.

16. Doherty, N. A., & Feeney, J. A. (2004). The composition of attachment networks throughout the adult years. *Personal Relationships, 11*, 469–488.

17. Efrati, J. (n.d.). *Drug dependence treatment: Training package.* Retrieved December 10, 2017, from https://www.unodc.org/ddt-training/treatment/general.htm.

18. Farrell, B. (2009). Mind, body, & soul. In "Collection development: Self-help audiobooks." *Library Journal, 134*(13), 36.

19. Følling, I. S., Solbjør, M., & Helvik, A. (2015). Previous experiences and emotional baggage as barriers to lifestyle change: A qualitative study of Norwegian Healthy Life Centre participants. *BMC Family Practice, 16*(1), 1–9. https://doi.org/10.1186/s12875-015-0292-z.

20. Frankl, V. E. (1963). *Man's search for meaning: An introduction to logotherapy*. New York: Washington Square Press.

21. Freud, S. (1995). Therapy and technique: "Wild" psycho-analysis. In P. Gay (Ed.), *The Freud reader*. London, England: Vintage Books.

22. Gates, R., & Hammond, R. (1993). When the music's over: A journey into schizophrenia (pp. 108–119). Sydney, Australia: University of UNE Press.

23. Gilman, S. L., King, H., Porter, R., Rousseau, G. S., & Showalter, E. (1993). *Hysteria beyond Freud*. Los Angeles: University of California Press.

24. Gray, S. (2011). *Competency-based assessments in mental health practice: Cases and practical application*. New Jersey, NJ: John Wiley & Sons.

25. Hall, C. (2016). Womanhood as experienced in childbirth: Psychoanalytic explorations of the body. *Psychoanalytic Social Work*, 1–18.

26. Hallstead, T. M. (2013). *Pygmalion's chisel: For women who are "never good enough"*. Retrieved from https://ebookcentral.proquest.com.

27. Jones, B. (2013). Becoming generative: Socialising influences recalled in life stories in late midlife. *Journal of Adult Development, 20*(3), 158–172.

28. Jung, C. (1960). On the nature of the psyche (1947/1954). In *Collected works* (Vol. 8, pp. 230–232).

29. Kitzinger, C., & Willmott, J. (2002). The thief of womanhood: Women's experience of polycystic ovarian syndrome. *Social Science & Medicine, 54*(3), 349–361. https://doi.org/10.1016/S0277-9536(01)00034-X.

30. Kolar, V. (1999). Learning parenting: Intergenerational influences. *Family Matters, 52*, 65–68.

31. Kosminsky, P., & Jordan, J. R. (2016). *Attachment-informed grief therapy: The clinician's guide to foundations and applications*. New York: Routledge.

32. Kottler, J. A. (2011). *The therapist's workbook: Self-assessment, self-care, and self-improvement exercises for mental health professionals*. Retrieved from https://ebookcentral.proquest.com

33. Lum, K. (2010, February 22). Schizophrenia – How it feels [Interview by B. Meyers]. Retrieved from https://www.youtube.com/watch?v=rWsYIoLZHYI.

34. Lynn, S., Green, J., Kirsch, I., Capafons, A., Lilienfeld, S., Laurence, J., & Montgomery, G. (2015). Grounding hypnosis in science: The "new" APA Division 30 definition of hypnosis as a step backward. *American Journal of Clinical Hypnosis, 57*(4), 390–401.

35. Mathis, R. [Ray]. (2017). *What you really need to do to keep fights and arguments from recurring* [LinkedIn page]. Retrieved December 12, 2017, from https://www.linkedin.com/groups/94332/94332-6341428139155087361?midToken=AQEvCFAP4D6-iA&trk=eml-b2_anet_digest_of_digests-group_discussions-18-discussion~subject&trkEmail=eml-b2_anet_digest_of_digests-group_discussions-18-discussion~subject-null-5l3idh~jbq2s5m1~4b-null-communities~group~discussion&lipi=urn%3Ali%3Apage%3Aemail_b2_anet_digest_of_digests%3BT7wjtNfyShOxEc9Tl8ueuw%3D%3D.

36. Mayo Clinic Staff. (2016, April 21). *Chronic stress puts your health at risk*. Retrieved December 12, 2017, from https://www.mayoclinic.org/healthy-lifestyle/stress-management/in-depth/stress/art-20046037.

37. McManus, T., & Nussbaum, J. (2011). Social support expectations and strategic ambiguity in parent–young adult child divorce-related stressor conversations. *Journal of Divorce & Remarriage, 52*(4), 244–270.

38. Meadows, G., Farrell, J., Fossey, E., Grigg, M., McDermott, F., & Singh, B. (2012). *Mental health in Australia: A collaborative community practice* (3rd ed.). Melbourne, Australia: Oxford University Press.

39. Mills, H., Reiss, N., & Dombeck, M. (2008, June 30). *Visualization and guided imagery techniques for stress reduction.* Retrieved November 27, 2017, from https://www.mentalhelp.net/articles/visualization-and-guided-imagery-techniques-for-stress-reduction.

40. Morris, T. (2014). *Mind, body, home: Transform your life one room at a time.* Minneapolis, MN: Llewellyn.

41. Moskowitz, A. (2009). Ego-fragmentation in schizophrenia: A severe dissociation of self-experience. In *Psychosis, trauma and dissociation* (pp. 51–64). Chichester, UK: John Wiley & Sons.

42. Myss, C. (2010). *The four archetypes of survival.* Archived from the original on May 29, 2012. Retrieved November 7, 2017.

43. National Council of Educational Research and Training. (2007). *Psychology: Textbook for class XI* (1st ed.). New Delhi, India: Author.

44. Norcross, J. C., & Guy, J. D. J. (2014). *Leaving it at the office: A guide to psychotherapist self-care.* Retrieved from https://ebookcentral.proquest.com.

45. Okken, R. (2012). *The liberating power of emotions.* Huntsville, AR: Ozark Mountain Publishing.

46. Orkibi, H., Azoulay, B., Regev, D., & Snir, S. (2017). Adolescents' dramatic engagement predicts their in-session productive behaviours: A psychodrama change process study. *The Arts in Psychotherapy, 55*, 46–53.

47. Perls, F., Hefferline, G., & Goodman, P. (1951). *Gestalt therapy*. New York, NY: [Publisher not specified].

48. Progoff, I. (1953). *Jung's psychology and its social meaning* (pp. 76–77). [Place of publication not specified].

49. Pyun, Y. (2015). Creating past-life identity in hypnotic regression. *International Journal of Clinical and Experimental Hypnosis, 63*(3), 365–372.

50. Rolfes, S. R., & Whitney, E. (2013). *Understanding nutrition*. Boston, MA: Cengage Learning.

51. Salman, S. (2008). The creative psyche: Jung's major contributions. In Young-Eisendrath & Dawson (Eds.), *Cambridge companion*. [Publisher not specified].

52. Schlotterbeck, K. (2003). *Living your past lives: The psychology of past-life regression*. Bloomington, IN: iUniverse.

53. Sebelis, S. (2011). Reflecting on relaxation. *Journal of the Australian Traditional-Medicine Society, 17*(2), 45–48.

54. Segal, R. A. (1999). *Theorizing about myth*. Amherst, MA: University of Massachusetts Press.

55. Selby, E. C., Shaw, E. J., & Houtz, J. C. (2005). The creative personality. *The Gifted Child Quarterly, 49*(4), 300–314, 356–357. Retrieved from http://ezproxy.navitas.com/login?url=https://search-proquest-com.ezproxy.navitas.com/docview/212081967?accountid=137399.

56. Singh, H. P. (2015, February 2). *Progress notes* [PowerPoint slides]. Retrieved December 12, 2017, from https://www.slideshare.net/RakeshVermatheboss/progress-notes-44191750.

57. Skovholt, T. M., & Trotter-Mathison, M. J. (2011). *The resilient practitioner: Burnout prevention and self-care strategies for counselors, therapists, teachers, and health professionals* (2nd ed.). Hoboken, NJ: Taylor and Francis.

58. Slater, C. L. (2003). Generativity versus stagnation: An elaboration of Erikson's adult stage of human development. *Journal of Adult Development, 10*(1), 53–65.

59. Solc, V. (2016, October 14). *Father archetype*. Retrieved January 2, 2018, from http://www.therapyvlado.com/english/father-archetype.

60. Stern, V. (2015). The fall and rise of subliminal messaging. *Scientific American Mind, 26*(5), 16–17.

61. Sternberg, E., Critchley, S., Gallagher, S., & Raman, V. (2011). A self-fulfilling prophecy: Linking belief to behaviour. *Annals of the New York Academy of Sciences, 1234*(1), 83–97. https://doi.org/10.1111/j.1749-6632.2011.06184.x.

62. Thompson, K. L., Hannan, S. M., & Miron, L. R. (2014). Fight, flight, and freeze: Threat sensitivity and emotion dysregulation in survivors of chronic childhood maltreatment. *Personality and Individual Differences, 69*, 28.

63. Van Biema, D. (1996). Of the soul: Combining medical advice with Indian metaphysics, Deepak Chopra has thrived, telling Americans of a place where spirit and body interact. *Time, 147*(26), 64.

64. Vitti, A. (2015, December 7). Is this set of emotions blocking your fertility? Retrieved December 20, 2017, from https://www.floliving.com/emotional-fertility-blocks.

65. von Franz, M. L. (1978). Man and his symbols. In C. G. Jung (Ed.). London, UK: [Publisher not specified].

66. Walker, J. (2010). *Complete mental health: The go-to-guide for clinicians and patients*. New York, NY: W. W. Norton & Company.

67. Wareham, J. (1998). Self-sabotage: Executive intelligence – Achievers' tendency to destroy themselves. *Across the Board, 35*(10), 49–50.

68. Willett, C., Anderson, E., & Meyers, D. (1999, June 28). *Feminist perspectives on the self*. Retrieved November 2, 2017, from https://plato.stanford.edu/entries/feminism-self.

'The gateways to wisdom and knowledge are always open.'

Louise Hay